OUTSMARTING STRESS

Biblical Principles for
Handling Life's Pressures

Richard Koole, Ed.D.

with
Raymond Schafer

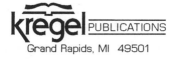

kregel PUBLICATIONS

Grand Rapids, MI 49501

Cover & book design: Alan G. Hartman

Library of Congress Cataloging-in-Publication Data

Koole, Richard Steven.

Outsmarting stress: biblical principles for handling life's pressures / Richard Koole.
     p.   cm.
   Includes bibliographical references and index.
   1. Stress (Psychology)—Religious aspects—Christianity. 2. Christian life—1960–   I. Title.
BV4501.2.K575   1993   248.8'6—dc20   92-23983
                                               CIP

ISBN 0-8254-3044-5 (pbk.)

1 2 3 4 5 6 Printing/Year 97 96 95 94 93

Printed in the United States of America

■■■■■■■■■■■■■■

DEDICATION

]   To Carolyn   [

CONTENTS

1
......■■■■■■■■■■...

HURRICANE WATCH

Recently a picture of Thelma Bellow appeared in newspapers across the country: She had just won ten million dollars through the "McMillions" giveaway sponsored by McDonald's. Unfortunately, she already had the check in hand when it was discovered that Mrs. Bellow had a daughter who was employed by McDonald's. She was declared ineligible and informed she couldn't claim the ten million dollars. You think you've got stress in your life—Thelma Bellow held a check for ten million dollars and no one would cash it!

WAITING FOR THE BIOPSY

There are many times in life when we experience stress. The doctor has taken a biopsy and you're anxiously awaiting the results. On Friday your boss announces that he wants to talk with you first thing Monday morning, and your stomach is tied up in knots all weekend. Your daughter has just started to drive; it's well past midnight now and she's not home with the car yet. You don't know where she is, and your mind is racing with unspeakable fears.

Your husband is growing progressively colder and you can't figure out why, so you live under a daily cloud of despair. You're three months behind on your bills and the bill collectors are harassing you now and demanding payment. You feel like running and hiding.

What should we do when life hurls these stressful situations at us?

In many cases, before we can respond *mentally*, our bodies react *physically*. Completely apart from our control, strange changes hit our bodies in reaction to life's stresses. Not only do

7

we experience a sudden rush of adrenaline, but doctors tell us that our muscles tighten in preparation for action. Sugar begins flowing into our blood system to provide a quick burst of power. Our breathing quickens as more oxygen is pumped through our blood to our muscles. A sudden slowdown in digestion may cause our stomach to ache as the blood pumps oxygen to our brain and muscles. Digestion is given a lower priority during stressful times, and our appetite is quickly lost. Our skin may feel cold as the blood is rerouted and sent to the muscles. This causes the skin to look pale and our extremities to feel cold. The pupils of the eyes dilate to allow better vision. The heart speeds up as blood is pumped at an increased rate through the body.

If the stress which triggered these reactions is relieved, our body soon returns to normal. If the situation continues, however, problems more severe or permanent may develop. For the sake of our mental, physical, and spiritual health we *must* learn how to recognize and minimize harmful stress in our lives.

However, we also need to realize that not all stress is bad, and that not all stress can or should be avoided. When brought under control, certain kinds of stress can provide us with a tremendous amount of productive energy. If we learn to harness such stresses we can redirect that productive energy into a wholesome force in our lives.

MORE THAN JUST A BREEZE

One of the most destructive forces on earth is a hurricane. A hurricane develops from narrow regions of low pressure called trade winds. Depending on the speed of these winds, tropical depressions can give birth to mighty hurricanes. The winds and the rain combined with the force of the sea produce huge waves that rise far above normal and cause severe flooding. A storm surge can be especially destructive if it happens at high tide. When the hurricane moves over land, strong winds and heavy rains may batter the area for several days or longer. Even after the winds decrease, the heavy rains continue.

During the hurricane season, meteorologists keep a close watch on the oceans. They also examine satellite pictures of the area and collect other vital information in order to forecast where a hurricane will hit and how strong it will be. Scientists have learned that the ability to minimize the damage done by a hurricane is predicated on *early detection*. If they can spot a tropical depression forming, they can better prepare people to survive its power.

Like a hurricane, stress will blow into our lives with tremendous force and untold potential for destruction. And also like a hurricane, *the ability to detect stress as it forms* is crucial to survival. Everyday stress from schedules, mundane jobs, and illness can literally blow us apart.

PERSONAL WEATHER FORECASTING

However, this type of stress need not be out of our control. We can do our own "weather forecasting" and know when these low-pressure areas are developing. We need to discover how to harness the winds of stress in order to push us forward rather than blow us away.

Dr. Roger Ritfal, Dean of the University of New Hampshire School of Health and Human Services, said regarding stress, "Everyone says stress is bad, but if you think of stress as energy, it's all in how you manage it. Stress can be the driving force that helps people reach their goals. Without a touch of stress in their lives, people wouldn't get anything done. The trick is finding the optimum where there is enough stress to avoid complacency, but not so much that it causes burnout."

Dr. Ritfal wasn't the first to point out this fact. In the Bible God tells us that stress is a necessary part of living. At times it is associated with the suffering promised the Christian in Philippians 1:29: "To you it has been granted on behalf of Christ, not only to believe in Him, but also to suffer for His sake."

But even though God tells us that *some* suffering is unavoidable, He warns us not to bring *self-inflicted* suffering on ourselves. This type of suffering will have no reward or benefit from God. Instead, we pay for it but receive nothing in return except tears, depression, and loss of joy. In this book we will show how to avoid unnecessary stress and harness the hurricanes in our lives.

TROPICAL DEPRESSIONS

Tropical depressions develop with the added velocity of the trade winds. As such winds of stress build in our own lives we need to be on the alert for bad weather ahead. In Ephesians 5 and 6 God lists eight areas of life in which these "tropical depressions" can form: 1) our health, 2) our relationship with the Holy Spirit, 3) our marriage, 4) our children, 5) our job, 6) our finances, 7) our defense against Satan, and 8) our thought life.

Ephesians 5:15,16 says, "See then that you walk circumspectly, not as fools but as wise, redeeming the time, because the days are evil. Therefore do not be unwise, but understanding what the will of the Lord is." Improper watchfulness in these areas of life can bring pain, frustration, and disaster.

To walk *circumspectly* means to watch accurately or carefully where we step. Let me illustrate what this means by sharing a time when I had to walk *circumspectly* on a golf course.

RATTLESNAKE RIDGE

As much as I enjoy playing the game of golf, I detest having to pay for new golf balls. They can be lost with any wild swing of the golf club . . . which happens to me more than I like! Recently I was playing a local golf course which had a steep hill surrounded by a barbed-wire fence. Many errant shots have landed in the heavy weeds on the hill, and attached to the fence were signs warning, "DO NOT ENTER . . . RATTLESNAKES. DANGER."

One day as I searched through the weeds on "Rattlesnake Ridge" I nearly stepped on a full-grown rattlesnake. It was coiled, rattling, and ready to strike. Fortunately I saw him in time and dodged out of the way. However, rather than cease my quest for free golf balls after such a scare, I continued on until all my pockets could hold no more golf balls. But I can assure you that I walked circumspectly—I took great care as I placed each step!

I learned that walking circumspectly not only means to be careful where we step but to watch and listen for *danger signs*— storm alerts warning us to seek protection.

STORM COMING: OPPORTUNITY AHEAD!

Ephesians 5:16 says, "Redeeming the time because the days are evil." The word *redeeming* means to rescue from loss. There are two Greek words for time, one emphasizing *chronological* time (as in days, hours, and months) and the other emphasizing opportunity. The word for *opportunity* is used here, alerting us to rescue our opportunities from loss.

The trade winds have blown, and tropical depressions are evident; a storm is approaching. Our lives are swirling with the winds of change and the rains of discouragement and fear; we're starting to feel out of control. How can we redeem ourselves in such a storm? As Earl Nightingale has said, "Where there is danger, there lurks opportunity. Where there is opportunity, there lurks danger. The two are inseparable; they go together." Reginald Mansel added, "A pessimist is one who makes difficulties of his opportunities. An optimist is one who makes opportunities out of his difficulties."

As we maneuver through the storms of our life we need to consider the difficulties we face to discover if they are just opportunities in disguise. Is God trying to develop our faith and reveal His strength by guiding us through the wind and the rain? Would we really want to miss knowing the reason for this journey?

The most crucial key to surviving a storm lies in *how we respond to it.* I am convinced that life is 10 percent what happens to us and 90 percent how we respond to it. Mark 4:35-41 describes a storm that caused the disciples to fear for their lives. As they were crossing the Sea of Galilee in their small fishing boat, a great storm of wind arose, and the waves beat against their boat. Jesus was asleep in the lower part of the boat, and in their fear they woke Him asking: "Teacher, do You not care that we are perishing?" Without any other action He spoke the simple words "Peace, be still "—and the wind ceased and the water calmed. In response to their reaction to the storm Jesus replied, "Why are you so fearful? How is it that you have no faith?" Even though these men had enjoyed the experience of walking day by day with Jesus Himself, they had not grasped His power and hope for their lives.

Just as Jesus told His disciples to let peace control them, His hope for us is the same today: We need to view the storms of our lives with less fear and more faith. A mature Christian is not one who has necessarily *done* great things but one who has *endured* great things. Malcolm Muggeridge expanded this theme when he stated, "Contrary to what might be expected, I look back on experiences that at the time seemed especially desolating and painful with particular satisfaction. Indeed, I can say with complete truthfulness that everything that I have learned in my 75 years in this world, everything that has truly enhanced my experience, has been through affliction and not happiness."

Although we enjoy the calm seas in life, it is *during the storms* that we find out what we're really made of. By navigating through the storms we learn the skills we need to equip us to face them again another day.

DECEPTIVE TRANQUILLITY

In the center of the hurricane lies an area of seeming peace and calm. This "eye of the storm" is surrounded by a wall of clouds which divide it from the fierce winds and rain of the rest of the hurricane. It is easy to be deceived by the peace and calm. A novice might think that the storm was over as this calm passed over him, but he would soon discover to his dismay that this temporary quiet was only an alert that the remaining fury of the storm was soon to follow.

In our lives we can be so deceived by the periods of calm and peace that we settle into complacency. This kind of peace is not the abiding confidence that God is able to control the winds and storms in our life but rather a confidence based on thinking that the storm will happen in someone *else's* life and not our own.

Everything seems so under control in our life. We coast along enjoying a job we have held for years. We know all the people we work with and who live near us. We are comfortable financially and are surrounded by family and friends who love us. Added to the previous comforts is the knowledge that our health is good and the future looks rosy.

HURLED INTO THE WIND

And then, when we least expect it, we are hurled out from the placid eye of the storm and into the raging winds that surround us. Perhaps we get fired or relocated, much to the dismay of our family. Without warning we are forced to leave the security of our home, family, and friends. Perhaps our health deteriorates due to neglect, illness, or age. We may find ourselves feeling deeply depressed, not understanding why or how we were blown so far from the calm.

The question now becomes, How will we respond to these changes in our life? Will we become *bitter* or *better*? We can allow ourselves to be blown helplessly along with the strong winds of stress and frustration, or we can be drawn through the storm with the determination to let it strengthen us. It is during such times of trial that we realize our true need for God's help.

It is no coincidence that when a Christian starts to become comfortable, God sends the winds of change, for He knows the value of storms in our lives. First Corinthians 10:13 tells us, "No temptation has overtaken you except such as is common to man; but God is faithful, who will not allow you to be tempted beyond what you are able, but with the temptation will also make the way of escape, that you may be able to bear it."

As the winds and storms blow across our lives God is there . . . and aware! We must only remember that our growth comes through *the experience of the storm* and not while we are safely anchored in calm waters.

PAIN WITH A PURPOSE

Suffering and trials also prepare us to serve others. I learned this lesson personally when I had major back surgery several years ago. Until that time I had never been in the hospital except to have my tonsils removed as a child. But with the back surgery I quickly developed a new understanding and empathy for those who suffer medical problems. Now when I encounter someone with a serious back problem, there is experience supporting my answers.

If you are presently going through suffering, it is not because God is out to get you; remember that Christ also experienced pain and suffering while He was on earth. It was in God's wisdom and plan for Jesus to have these experiences, so that He could have even greater empathy for the human race and for our suffering.

Just as Jesus experienced suffering with a purpose, so do we. God can use our pain, illness, and loss to help others. We can encourage others to grow with us by sharing the victory of our suffering.

One night a family from our church called. They were heartbroken because of a tragedy that had just happened to one of their children. I didn't understand at the time why God would allow a crisis like this to strike such a fine family or how it could be used to help others; it seemed so unfair.

However, in the days that followed I became highly impressed with their strength as they rallied around each other and God. Within a week I received another phone call, this time from another Christian family that was much less mature in the Lord but had just experienced the same kind of tragedy. I never would have expected to face this problem again in my ministry, let alone within the same week, but here it was. Although I didn't know how to personally relate to this father and mother, I knew of a family that could. The first couple was able to share with the less mature family the strength that God had provided for them. Out of their tragedy they became better prepared to serve others in need.

LIVING WHAT WE CLAIM

Missionary B. W. Woods experienced what seemed like the ultimate tragedy while on the mission field. Because of disease and the lack of proper medical attention, his wife and only child died. He was left alone on the mission field with the natives watching his every move. "They saw him walk to the graves of his wife and child in a quiet and stately manner. They sensed in his grief a note of hope and victory. One was heard to say, 'I don't know about his religion, or the Christ he serves, but I do know that I like the way he buries his dead. There is a difference between his sorrow and ours. We shriek with horror and anguish, and we have no hope, but this man acts as if he knows where his dead wife and child are going.'"

I've stood at the hospital bed of many a Christian, both young and old, as they have felt life slip away and death draw near. I have benefited from the victory they have proclaimed while preparing to meet their Savior. I can honestly say that nobody dies like a Christian.

On the other hand, I have also been with the unsaved as they have faced death. They have no hope, and it shows. Christians are different: They know where they're going, and it shows. We know that the moment our last breath is taken we will be ushered into the presence of our Lord and Savior.

When sorrows strike the believer, even as the natives who observed the calm assurance of missionary B. W. Woods, the world is watching. We face the same grief as the unsaved: We lose jobs and agonize over our children; we suffer physical and emotional setbacks; we live with the knowledge of a terminal illness. What the world wants to know is, Do we live what we claim? Is our faith real?

The greatest gift a Christian can share with the world is hope. There was a song written years ago which stated that love was the world's greatest need, yet without *hope*, even love struggles. When the unsaved see strength in the midst of the storms in our lives, they are drawn to that strength because it offers hope. It is then that we can share with them the true source of our strength . . . Jesus Christ.

REMOVING THE WEEDS

The Bible is very clear concerning Satan's attempts to infiltrate the church: Where there is wheat there are also tares or weeds. Have you ever noticed how the weeds in your yard look almost like grass when they are mowed right along with the real thing? Unfortunately, the weeds that grow right along with the grass have the potential of overtaking and overpowering it. Soon there are just as many weeds as grass, and the lawn isn't the same anymore. Unless we get rid of the weeds by removing them by the roots, they will soon be in charge instead of us.

In the church the wheat is in danger of being taken over in the same way. The weeds that Satan plants in the church—those people who are not really serving God but appear to be—can be difficult to detect. Satan doesn't plant the ugly, thorny variety; he selects the hearty, nice-looking ones. The wheat—the true servants of Christ—need to be watched over and nourished with good doctrinal teaching. The tares become more evident when exposed by the Word of God on a regular basis. Without the removal of the tares, the wheat will not be able to produce the harvest it should.

This process of removing Satan's weeds from the church can bring great suffering to God's wheat. Fortunately, the fires that burn off the weeds purify the church at the same time. William Penn used to say, "No pain, no gain; no thorns, no throne; no gall, no glory; no cross, no crown. We must remember that when things are tough, it is the rubbing and tumbling of stones against abrasives that brings out their luster and shine. Talents rise out of adversities, not prosperous circumstances. Kites rise only when going against the wind."

WHAT IS YOUR THORN?

If there was ever a man with a reason to be puffed up with pride, it was the apostle Paul. What extraordinary gifts and blessings he experienced! Yet God allowed Satan to send Paul a messenger, a thorn in the flesh. In 2 Corinthians 12:8,9 we read that Paul prayed three times for God to take away the physical thorn in his flesh, but each time the answer Paul received was no.

How would you have responded to being turned down in triplicate? Listen as Paul gives his response: "Lest I should be exalted above measure by the abundance of the revelations, a thorn in the flesh was given to me, a messenger of Satan to buffet me, lest I be exalted above measure. Concerning this thing I pleaded with the Lord three times that it might depart from me. But He said to me, 'My grace is sufficient for you, for My strength is made perfect in weakness.' Therefore most gladly I will rather boast in my infirmities, that the power of Christ may rest upon me. Therefore I take pleasure in infirmities, in reproaches, in needs, in persecutions, in distresses, for Christ's sake. For when I am weak, then I am strong" (1 Corinthians 12:7-10).

Paul could take pleasure in his weaknesses because he knew they would keep his pride under control. He also knew that "God resists the proud, but gives grace to the humble" (James 4:6).

Perhaps God has delivered a messenger into your life. These messengers bring pain, loneliness, depression, false guilt, and distraction into our lives. We struggle with them daily. If we, like Paul, can see these trials for what they are, they can become personal barometers signaling a change in our spiritual climate. The suffering they bring is not enjoyable, but it can protect us from the harm that pride can inflict.

TYRANT IN YOUR LIFE

Charles Hummel wrote about something called "the tyranny of the urgent" which tends to invade our lives all the time. While sitting down for dinner with the family the phone rings; you can almost count on it. And it's difficult to not answer it, because the ringing sounds urgent. But is that call important enough to sacrifice the fellowship of our family? We tend to surrender our time to things which claim to be urgent without first weighing their importance. We end up taking care of things that merely *seem* urgent while shoving aside those things which really *are* urgent.

A young friend of mine was called to pastor his first church. He was a good man and had a supportive wife, but this new church was notorious for its problems. However, if anyone could turn this church around, it was this couple. So they went to work with unbridled dedication and enthusiasm.

After several months they were struggling with the same problems which had caused their predecessors to leave, and were getting burned out. As this young man spent more and more time trying to solve the seemingly urgent problems of other people, slowly his own marriage began to crumble. At this point a friend sat down with him and explained what was happening: He was being ruled by the tyranny of the urgent. He thought his number one priority was to get the church back into shape when in fact his highest priorities should have been first to God, then to his family, and finally to the church. He could leave the church and find another place to minister, but if he lost his wife, he lost everything.

Sometimes we behave as if our job is the most important thing in our life. We are willing to risk our marriage over it. Other times we are so preoccupied with finances that we gamble our relationship with our children. We spend so much time pursuing money that we don't even have time to spend it. We get so busy that we forget which things ought to be the non-negotiables of life.

WHAT IS NEGOTIABLE?

Gordon MacDonald addressed the non-negotiables when he wrote, "They never screamed out immediately when ignored. I could neglect my spiritual disciplines, for example, and God did not seem to shout loudly about it. I could make it just fine for a while. And when I did not allocate time for the family, Gail and the children were generally understanding and forgiving—often more so than certain church members who demanded instant response and attention. And when I set study aside things could be ignored for a while without adverse consequences. And that is why they were so often crowded out when I did not budget for them in advance. Other less important issues had a way of wedging them aside week after week. Tragically, if they are neglected too long—when family, rest, and spiritual disciplines are finally noticed—it is often too late for adverse consequences to be avoided."

The time we spend with the Lord must be a non-negotiable relationship, yet when we encounter busy days we often sacrifice our time with the Lord. It doesn't seem to hurt us at first. As a matter of fact, we may go for weeks without spending time with God and still appear to survive. This is also true in our marriages.

We fail to spend meaningful time with our spouse and seem to get away with it. However, if we don't go to work for three days, there will be an immediate crisis.

Although the true non-negotiables don't seem to scream for immediate attention, they will exact a much higher price when neglected. Eventually our world crashes in as we realize (often too late) that our relationships at home and with Jesus Christ are far more important than those things which appeared to be so urgent at the time.

God can use times of suffering, illness, and isolation to allow us to examine the priorities in our life. When we are laid flat on our back physically or emotionally we start to see *who*, and not *what*, is important in life. We spend time with the Lord and are reminded of the joy we have missed. We spend time with our family and realize how precious this relationship truly is.

NOT JUST THE LIGHT THREADS

When Christians go through suffering but gain victory by it, Satan's attempts become foiled and he is perplexed. In the book of Job, Satan and God were gathered around the throne, and Satan was boasting about the people on earth he thought he could cause to fall, when God said, "Consider Job." (He must have been confident that Job would not fall under stress.) Satan responded by saying, "Of course he honors You—look at all You have given him." To this God replied, "Go ahead—you can do anything but kill him." So Satan immediately went to work on Job. He took his servants, his flocks, and even his children. The only people Satan did not take from Job's life were his nagging wife and his three friends who eventually turned on him.

Job had been called by God to endure unusual suffering victoriously in order to show future generations the outcome of those who place their complete trust in God. Every time a Christian endures suffering and is able to continue to praise God's name, Satan suffers a battle loss of major proportions.

Our lives, like a fine tapestry, need both dark as well as light threads to produce the proper results. Without the dark threads the picture would lack depth and color; *with* the dark threads the tapestry becomes magnificent!

2

HEALTH ON THE BRINK

"Do not be drunk with wine, in which is dissipation, but be filled with the Spirit" (Ephesians 5:18). God declares that we have a *choice* about who and what controls our lives. He knows we will have opportunities in life to be exposed to many outside influences that can affect what goes on inside our bodies. How we choose to handle these will impact not only our lives but the lives of those around us.

BODY SIGNALS

Our bodies often indicate the presence of stress long before we can acknowledge it with our minds. Short-term symptoms of stress include headaches and trouble falling or staying asleep. Other symptoms include vomiting, diarrhea, or loss of appetite. Daily decisions and the ability to concentrate can become difficult. Unexplained fatigue may make it hard for us to keep up with our normal schedule. We can place the blame for these symptoms on many illnesses (and they should be explored), but we often fail to deal with the *stress* in our lives that may be the true culprit.

There is a very real connection between daily emotional stresses and the physical problems that result. If we fail to find relief from severe stress, we risk more serious medical problems, including high blood pressure, strokes, and heart disease. Allergies, skin disorders, and asthma can intensify if our stress level is not decreased. Because our nervous system becomes more sensitive while under stress, we may experience physical pain throughout our body without apparent cause. Doctors tell us that infection may develop and spread when the long-term effects of stress have lowered our immunities.

SPIRIT-FILLED HEALTH

One of our highest priorities should be the proper care of our health. When we take care of our bodies properly we find that the effect of stress in our lives is greatly reduced.

Proper care of our body is biblically important because of the involvement of the Holy Spirit; the last part of Ephesians 5:18 states, "Be filled with the Spirit." This admonition should make us fearful of doing anything that could harm our health. If we choose to fill our lives with influences that rob the Holy Spirit of His rightful dwelling place and control, we invite the stressful effects that will result.

First Corinthians 6:19 tells us, "Your body is the temple of the Holy Spirit. " God instructed the Jewish people to take meticulous care of the earthly temple prior to its destruction in A.D. 70 because it was the dwelling place of God. That temple has long since been destroyed, but in a real sense there is still a temple of God, and that temple is our body. Because of this our body is not ours to do with as we please; we need to let it shine for God by removing any obstacles that get in the way of God's glory.

What are such obstacles? Here are five of them that bring shame to God and ruination to ourselves.

ALCOHOL . . . WASTER OF DREAMS

The statistics on the use of alcohol in the United States are alarming. Each year 80,000 people die because of alcoholism! That's 30,000 more people than we lost during the seven-year conflict in Vietnam. In addition to the fact that as many as 90 percent of all highway fatalities are alcohol-related, two out of three drownings result from alcohol abuse. Eight out of ten fatal fires in the home are caused by drunkenness. Half of all violent crimes accompany alcohol abuse.

The issue at stake here is *control*: "Do not be drunk with wine, in which is dissipation, but be filled with the Spirit" (Ephesians 5:18). When anything has control of our minds, it will control our bodies also. God says that we will be dissipated when alcohol controls us. The word in Greek for dissipation means "to be wasted." This same word is used in Luke 15 to refer to the Prodigal Son, who dissipated or wasted his inheritance from his father.

Drunkenness is the waster of dreams: It wastes marriages; it wastes children as alcoholic parents rob children of their childhood; it wastes good jobs; it wastes tremendous personal potential. "Friedeman Bach, the most gifted son of the great German composer Johann Sebastian Bach, went to pieces through drink. Michael Haydn, the younger brother of Joseph Haydn, and hardly less gifted, was ruined by drink. Franz Schubert became an inveterate wine drinker and died in his early thirties. Robert Schumann's drunkenness led to a nervous breakdown. After the death of his wife, Rembrandt (then 36) became an alcoholic. Said Upton Sinclair, 'I call drink the greatest trap that life has set for the feet of genius!'"

We read daily in the papers about lives being wasted because of drunken drivers. I just put down a newspaper in which I read about the charges against a person accused of killing three people while driving under the influence of alcohol. Drunkenness can cause the waste of entire families—the lives of both the alcoholic and his victims.

Recently a man from our church called me from jail. He had gotten drunk and beaten his wife. (Yes, it happens to Christians too.) Anyone who allows himself to be controlled by alcohol will experience waste in his or her life. When we talk with the children of alcohol-abusers we witness the scars of humiliation, neglect, injury, and loss that they will wear for the rest of their lives.

The waste is also carried to the workplace. Employers tell of no-shows, sloppy performance, and injuries on the job due to alcohol abuse.

When people reach the point in their lives where the bottom has fallen out from under them, they often try to blame everyone and everything other than where the real guilt lies. Even God gets blamed for the tragedies that befall them, despite the fact that He has given clear biblical guidance about controlling our lives.

FOOD . . . TOO MUCH OF A GOOD THING

Every night at about 11 I fight a noble battle: I get the bedtime urge for a piece of toast smothered in peanut butter and jelly! I'm thankful that food can be so tasty and affect our health and duration of life, but it can also diminish our ability to serve God.

Gluttony, or the lack of control in eating, can be just as damaging as alcohol abuse. God tells us that both are sins. Scripture often refers to gluttony in the same breath as drunkenness. Proverbs 23:21 says, "The drunkard and the glutton will come to poverty." Matthew 11:19 speaks of "a gluttonous man and a winebibber." Both of these abuses show that submission to the control of an outside influence can result in poverty of the body, soul, and spirit.

Our bodies are much like fine-tuned automobiles. They may vary as far as model year and design, and they may serve somewhat different purposes, but they all need proper care and fuel. Even though they seem to run fairly well on inadequate care for awhile, eventually they start to show the signs of improper maintenance.

As the years accumulate, we are much more likely to hear, "Well, at your age you can expect to have problems" every time we ask a doctor why we don't feel so good. It is a fact of life that we are all growing older and that aging takes its toll on everybody. We are told by God the Great Physician as well as by human physicians to take care of our bodies lest we rush the aging process and magnify the stress in our lives. Since there are only a few areas of stress in our lives that we can control, we need to work hard at reducing stress in these areas. The quality and quantity of food intake is one of these areas.

Improper care of our bodies will limit not only our lifestyle but also our service for God. For example, we tend to shy away from life when we are embarrassed by our weight; it distracts our attention from what we are called to be and do. We tend to become *self*-conscious instead of *Christ*-conscious. The body of the overweight individual not only suffers, but the body of Christ also suffers when he or she fails to use the spiritual gifts given to help the church.

SOLVING THE WEIGHT PROBLEM

Statistics show that two years after beginning a diet most people weigh at least as much as they did prior to starting the diet. Usually there is an initial loss of weight, but defeat occurs as people fail to follow through. They tire of the regimentation and drop off the diet, then gain more weight than if they hadn't gone on the diet in the first place. I don't say this to discourage you, but to show you the value of a better alternative.

The people who have the most success in losing weight and keeping it off are those who recognize the problem of overweight as a *battle of the spirit*. They have learned to view gluttony as a sin, recognizing it as a distraction keeping them from full concentration on the purpose that God has for their lives.

I know preachers who cannot preach on the subject of gluttony, for obvious reasons. As a preacher myself I have to realize that there are areas on which I must preach that I am dealing with in my own life. To allow sins which are preventable to control me to the extent that they limit my ministry would be a serious sin. This keeps me constantly alert to maintain the freedom I need to preach the Word of God without apology.

I have dealt with a number of couples experiencing marital problems in which one of the partners was considerably overweight. I have learned to recognize this as a very dangerous situation. Red flags are flying! In nearly every case, the person who has worked to maintain a pleasing physical appearance feels defrauded. In such relationships infidelity is often the result.

A person who is overweight runs the risk of losing his or her spouse. The partner may appear to be loyal, but resentment may be building deep inside. After all, he or she married a physically attractive person who no longer seems to care that it matters to the spouse how he or she looks. Many times the end result is divorce.

Soon after the divorce, diets are often started and there is a revamping of the wardrobe. But the best time to start that diet should be *before* the divorce. We need to keep our self-respect and have the knowledge that we are in the very best shape we can be for our spouses, ourselves, our families, and our God. When we are at our best, we are in control of the things that can distract us from serving God instead of letting them control us.

BENT BOWS AND SHARP TOOLS

There was a man who spent 30 years preparing for three years of intense work. Even though the importance of His work would change the world forever, He was careful to make time for refreshment and to renew His focus on what was to come. This man was Jesus. In Mark 6:31 He told his disciples, "Come aside by yourselves to a deserted place and rest a while." Jesus created the human body and knew its need for rest.

Jesus gave us a living example of the need for rest. He grew weary of the constant stress of the crowds and the demands they made on Him. As every archer knows, a bow cannot always be in a bent position without breaking or losing its effectiveness.

Charles Haddon Spurgeon said, "Rest time is not waste time. It is economy to gather fresh strength. Look at the mower in the summer's day, with so much to cut down before the sun sets. He pauses in his labor—is he a sluggard? He looks for his stone, and begins to draw it up and down his scythe, with 'rink-a-tink—rink-a-tink—rink-a-tink.' Is it idle music . . . is he wasting precious moments? How much he might have mown while he has been ringing out those notes on his scythe! But he is sharpening his tool, and he will do far more when once again he gives his strength to those long sweeps which lay the grass down prostrate in rows before him. Even so, a little pause prepares the mind for greater service in the good cause."

Moses, Paul, and Peter all got away for rest. These great men of the faith knew their need for retreat. Are we stronger than they? I have heard men claim to be above the need for rest, only to hear later that they burned out. They ignored God's example and commands and paid for it in the currency of personal stress. Preachers who proclaim that they can't find time to get away from their churches must be doing something wrong (besides being a bad example to their congregation). They are overestimating the need for their presence while underestimating their need for rest. If pastors don't take time to refresh themselves, they will go stale on their congregations.

We need to have a change from the daily routine. Because my daily routine is mostly mental, I relax through strenuous physical exercise. It may involve running or fighting the pounding surf off the coast of Southern California. For those with other interests or physically tiring jobs, rest may mean spending a quiet day alone or doing something fun with their family. Whatever the form, the key is *change*.

TIRED WARRIORS OF THE ROAD

Have you observed the way some people try to relax while taking a summer vacation? They become "road warriors." Dad insists that the family rise no later than 5:00 a.m. While Dad is barking out instructions, Mom is trying to dress the kids and pour the cereal so they don't have to stop for breakfast on the road. Dad announces that they will drive until 8:30 p.m. Fifteen hours on the road, and heaven help the child who needs a pit stop!

After maintaining this kind of schedule for two hectic weeks, they limp back home with nerves frayed to the breaking point, and the children cry "mutiny" at the thought of ever going on vacation again!

Lee Iaccoca talked about vacations in his book *Iaccoca*. As he met with key executives who were leading 500-million-dollar divisions of his corporation, he asked them about their vacation plans. Some boasted that they were so busy they had no time to take a vacation. Iaccoca responded by questioning their importance to the corporation. "If you are in charge of a 500-million-dollar-a-year auto division, with all the planning and all the organization that accompanies that position, and you are not organized enough to schedule two weeks of vacation out of 52, I question whether you are competent to run your division. *Take a vacation.*"

The one-in-seven principle of rest applied even to the use of the land in the Old Testament. God commanded that every seventh year the land was to rest in order to prevent burnout. When the Jews ignored God's command for 490 years, God sent them into captivity in Babylon for 70 years, thereby giving the land rest for 70 years, or one-seventh of the 490 overworked years.

As with the land of Israel, we are sometimes forced by God into long periods of rest. This can happen, for example, when we suffer extended illness or unemployment. At such times we get our long-neglected physical and mental restoration.

Recently a friend of mine was laid off for a long period of time. During this period he reevaluated his old job and discovered that he really wanted to do something else. With the help of a supportive wife he went back to school and is now training for a job that will suit his personality and gifts much better. He is a happier man because of his unplanned captivity.

Work is a vital part of life, but if abused it can destroy us. We need to be in control of how work affects our lives, our homes, and our service to God. If everything focuses around our job, then trouble lurks around the corner. The ultimate pay we will receive will be in the form of destructive personal stress.

GUARANTEED TO DESTROY

We sometimes damage our lives with habits that are guaranteed to destroy. *Drugs* and *tobacco* fit into this category. I recently spoke with one of my relatives whose husband passed away some years ago. He and his four brothers died from either emphysema or lung cancer. All five brothers were heavy smokers who rolled their own cigarettes. My relative noted that when they began to smoke, doctors had not yet discovered all the dangers of tobacco.

Her husband was shocked when he found out that he had lung cancer and that it had been brought on by cigarette smoking. As he left the doctor's office he dumped the whole pack into the sewer and never smoked again, but it was too late. He and his wife were left to suffer the painful stress of facing death at the whims of an unmerciful disease.

Drugs also vie for control of our lives. "According to the National Association on Prenatal Addiction Research and Education, 375,000 drug-exposed children were born in the U.S.A. in 1987. Those exposed to crack cocaine run the risk of behavioral abnormalities, growth retardation, small head size, poor nutrition, and infection by sexually transmitted diseases. The pain that crack babies experience and the length of time it takes them to withdraw from the drug to which they are born addicted has been well publicized. Why then does a mother subject her child to such pain?"

The answer, pure and simple, is *lack of control*. The pregnant women addicted to crack are out of control. Addicts sell their possessions, barter their self-respect, lie, steal, and cheat to get the drugs their bodies crave. Impending motherhood does not change that awful reality. Peter B. Gemma Jr. adds, "If there were a cruelty rating in the gruesome statistics of the child abuse crisis, certainly inflicting pain and physical harm on unborn and newborn babies would have to be among the worst. Each day more than 1000 infants are brought into this world writhing in pain of dope addiction and facing frighteningly high mortality rates. Many of these precious little ones are suffering brain damage, blindness, seizures, and horrible deformities. Why is this happening right here in the U.S.A.? Simply because crack, coke and a variety of other incredibly dangerous drugs are being force-fed to developing babies . . . either through ignorance or criminal negligence . . . by their mothers during pregnancy."

These poor babies are born with a neurological deformity that will be with them for the rest of their lives. Schoolteachers tell us these kids are "bouncing off the walls" in their classrooms.

It is dangerous to abuse drugs for any reason. As Christian adults we need to make responsible choices in what we allow to affect or control our lives. We cannot afford the resulting stress that this form of abuse brings into our homes, churches, and jobs.

HOLY SWEAT

An article titled "Report Children Out of Shape" speaks about the poor physical condition of Western children. "Most of California's schoolchildren are physically unfit, and the problem may not improve anytime soon. A fitness test given to 917,404 fifth-, seventh-, and ninth-graders found that more than 75 percent of the children failed to meet minimum standards, according to the State Education Department. The majority of those tested were too slow at running or too weak to do pull-ups and sit-ups. More than one-third were fat."

These are our children, and we need to be concerned about them. Children often follow in the steps of their parents; are we setting a good example in this area of our lives?

Some of the positive benefits of exercise are that we feel better, sleep better, look better, and resist illness better. Exercise also strengthens our cardiovascular system and lifts our spirits. It can bring us to our very best and keep us there.

How can we make exercise the priority it should be in our lives? The answer is *consistency*. We need to make a commitment and stick with it. To do this, we need to find a method of exercise that we enjoy, because if we don't like it we won't stick with it. Sometimes exercise is more enjoyable if we share it with a friend. Besides enjoying companionship, we become accountable to someone. If we determine not to quit for at least three months, usually we can see and feel the benefit of the exercise, and then we won't want to quit.

Even more important is the benefit of exercise to our hearts. Some people work hard to build up their biceps, and that's good, but I've never heard of anyone dying because of a weak left bicep. Yet medical records show that one-fourth of all American males who died last year died from some form of heart disease. We need to concentrate on exercise that will strengthen our hearts!

Consistent daily exercise can prolong our life and preserve its quality. If we live longer and healthier lives, we can be much more productive in our service to God. We can better withstand the storms of life and still have reserve energy to serve God with our whole person. This becomes especially

important as we become older and have less control over what
happens to our bodies.

THE CALEB CHALLENGE

Caleb was one of the 12 spies sent by Moses into the Promised
Land. After seeing the land, he and Joshua declared that Israel
should go for it. They shared this confidence even after they had
surveyed the treacherous mountainous areas, the fortified walled
cities, and the fierce giants called Anakim. The ten other spies
didn't believe they could conquer all these obstacles, but Caleb
and Joshua believed that God would make it possible. Caleb
was 40 years old when he returned from surveying the land.

Because the people of Israel lacked the faith to obey God and
enter the land, He sentenced them to wander through the barren
Sinai Peninsula for more than 40 years. During this time all the
men who were over 20 years old at the time of the survey died,
and their bones littered the route of their journey. Only two men
from this older generation survived: Joshua and Caleb.

Forty-five years later Israel was finally preparing for the
conquest of the land. While the young warlords were deciding
who should attack which part of Canaan, an old warrior by the
name of Caleb moved to the front and proclaimed, "Behold, the
Lord has kept me alive, as He said, these forty-five years, ever
since the Lord spoke this word to Moses while Israel wandered
in the wilderness; and now, here I am this day, eighty-five years
old. As yet I am as strong this day as I was on the day that
Moses sent me; just as my strength was then, so now is my
strength for war, both for going out and for coming in. Now
therefore, give me this mountain" (Joshua 14:10-12).

Caleb demanded the most challenging terrain; he wanted the
mountains where the giants lived. That was also where the walled
cities and the chariots of iron were. Because of Caleb's faith, God
had preserved not only his life but also his physical strength.

We all need to take the "Caleb Challenge." I don't know how
long my life will be, but I do know that if I don't take care of
myself I will have neither as many years nor as much good
health as I should have in order to challenge the mountains and
giants in my way.

Let's not frustrate God's plans for us by needlessly abusing
our bodies. Instead, let's reach for the very best health that we
can get!

3

POWER ON THE INSIDE

Stress lurks around every corner in these times. We have a federal budget that doesn't come close to balancing, a national financial situation that has the stock market gyrating up and down, and a continuing Mideast crisis that never seems to end.

So where is God in these times? To understand where He is today, we need to look at the past habitations of God. We know He was resident with Israel in the Ark of the Covenant as the people crossed the Sinai wilderness on their way to the Promised Land.

THE DWELLING PLACE OF GOD

When a permanent temple was built, God dwelt in a place where His people could worship and approach Him. Upon the completion of Solomon's temple, God declared in 1 Kings 9:3-5, "I have heard your prayer and your supplication that you have made before Me; I have sanctified this house which you have built to put My name there forever, and My eyes and My heart will be there perpetually. Now if you walk before Me as your father David walked, in integrity of heart and uprightness, to do according to all that I have commanded you, and if you keep My statutes and My judgments, then I will establish the throne of your kingdom over Israel forever, as I promised David your father, saying, 'You shall not fail to have a man on the throne of Israel.'"

Solomon spared nothing in the construction of this dwelling place of God; most of the interior was covered with gold. He fulfilled the dream of his father David by erecting "an exalted house, and a place for You to dwell in forever" (1 Kings 8:13).

These verses show four unique qualities of this special building.

1. The temple had great value in both its cost and its purpose.
2. Solomon took meticulous care in both its design and construction because God was to inhabit it.
3. Though it was built by man, the temple was dedicated and given to God for His use.
4. Because it was God's house, there was no room for other gods in the temple. It was not to be defiled.

Along with most of the rest of the city, the temple in Jerusalem was destroyed in A.D. 70 by the Roman general Titus. Even though the building was destroyed, its inhabitant was not; God will always have a dwelling place. In His wisdom and grace God chose a new residence. Instead of dwelling in a single temple where only priests were allowed to approach Him, today God lives in many dwelling places where His children can worship and freely meet with Him. First Corinthians 6:19 says, "Do you not know that your body is the temple of the Holy Spirit who is in you, whom you have from God, and you are not your own?" God has chosen *our bodies* as His new residence.

WALKING TEMPLES

I am stricken with awe when I consider the full impact of this statement. It should instill the fear of God in us all. *We are walking, talking, working temples of God.* Just like Solomon's temple, we too have incredible value. At a price far more costly than gold, our purchase was made with the life of God's only Son, Jesus. We need to take meticulous care of our bodies in every way because the inhabitant within us is *God Himself*. Even though we were conceived by man, as Christians our bodies are not our own, but have been dedicated to God. We need to keep this center of worship as God's alone, not allowing other gods to control or defile us.

First Kings 9:6,7 is the final admonition of God at the dedication of Solomon's temple, and it speaks powerfully to us today: "If you or your sons at all turn from following Me, and do not keep My commandments and My statutes which I have set before you, but go and serve other gods and worship them, then I will cut off Israel from the land which I have given them; and this house which I have sanctified for My name I will cast out of my sight. Israel will be a proverb and a byword among all peoples."

If we choose to defile our bodies and minds, and to allow our service to go to anyone else but God, we become a displeasure in God's eyes, and our lives become a byword instead of a statement of God's power.

HALF-EMPTY OR FULLY FILLED?

The moment he is saved each Christian receives the Holy Spirit. This baptism of the Holy Spirit is permanent (Romans 8:9; 1 Corinthians 12:13). However, on any given day we have different degrees of filling of the Holy Spirit. In my own life there are times when I get careless in my spiritual walk and feel like I am half-empty and not properly prepared to serve Christ. I feel totally inadequate to battle with Satan. My temple shows little evidence of the filling of the Holy Spirit. On other days, when I have taken care to read my Bible and spend time talking to God in prayer, I am prepared for the warfare around me, and God's presence is evident within me.

Satan has a strong desire to control the lives of each of us. Even though the *indwelling* of the Spirit in us is permanent, the amount of His *filling* can change day by day and moment by moment. Nothing causes more stress in our lives than allowing Satan and his influences to defile us by letting him have access and control. When we let him gain ground the Holy Spirit cannot rule properly within our lives. The temple that God has sanctified becomes defiled, turning into a battleground for control. We rob God of His rightful dwelling place and severely hamper His ability to use us.

Ephesians 5:18-21 states, "Do not be drunk with wine, in which is dissipation, but be filled with the Spirit, speaking to one another in psalms and hymns and spiritual songs, singing and making melody in your heart to the Lord, giving thanks always for all things to God the Father in the name of our Lord Jesus Christ, submitting to one another in the fear of God." Our real victory over daily struggles and stress comes through the *filling of the Holy Spirit*. When we allow the Holy Spirit to control our lives, we achieve harmony with God and He then has the freedom to unleash incredible overcoming power within us.

THE GREATEST POWER IN THE WORLD

A. J. Gordon tells of an English gentleman who was viewing the Niagara whirlpool rapids when an American friend remarked,

"Come, and I'll show you the greatest unused power in the world." He led him to the foot of Niagara Falls and said, "There is the greatest unused power in the world." "Ah, no, my brother, not so," was the reply. "The greatest unused power in the world is the Holy Spirit of God!" The reason the power of the Holy Spirit is not being unleashed in churches across America today is that it is not being unleashed in the lives of individual Christians.

In 1 Peter 5:8 Satan is referred to as a roaring lion; he roams around stalking Christians like you and me, trying to destroy our potential usefulness to God. By defiling the temple of God, he makes us a mockery instead of a shrine to God's glory. We need to realize, "Greater is He that is in you than he that is in the world" (1 John 4:4). More than enough power rests within each of us, in the Person of the Holy Spirit, to overcome all the roaring lions awaiting us.

Nothing is more exciting than watching as the Holy Spirit demonstrates His power to bring the lost to Christ. This was revealed dramatically while Dr. Newman Hall was visiting Wales. One morning he arose early to join about 120 people from the town who had gathered on the summit of Snowden to view a grand sunrise. As the sun rose it became more spectacular than they could have imagined. As they marveled at the beauty of God's creation, Dr. Hall was invited to pray. A serene stillness swept over the people as he spoke to God. Tears streamed down their faces as he closed the prayer with a sincere "Amen" and descended the hill. Some time later he was informed that 40 people had come to know Christ because of his words. "But," responded Dr. Hall, "I didn't say a word to them—I only prayed." Said a friend in reply, "Yes, and more wonderful still, they didn't know a word you said, for none of them could speak English— only Welsh." When we fail to give the Holy Spirit the freedom to fill us we miss great opportunities for witness in our lives.

The Holy Spirit has the freedom to reach out to others in unique ways as we simply go about our normal daily walk. In his book *The Wind and the Spirit*, Vance Havner writes, "There is mystery, there is power, and we cannot chart the course of the Spirit. He is sovereign to do as He pleases, just as the wind blows where it wills. He did not use the same method or manner with Savonarola and Knox and Luther and Wesley and Moody. Just as there are hurricanes and zephyrs, so the Spirit storms and soothes. He speaks in a mighty tornado or the gentlest whisper. The Spirit did not work in the Reformation as He did in the Great Awakening. With Whitefield he blew in one fashion, with Moody in another. The Great Awakening was not like the Welsh Revival." When the Spirit goes to work we are privileged to experience the greatest power the world has ever seen!

ENGINES WITHOUT OIL

There has been much confusion about the doctrine of the Holy Spirit in the past few decades. Many evangelical churches have witnessed abuses of the doctrine and have become fearful of even talking about the Holy Spirit. A. W. Tozer addressed this problem when he wrote, "The doctrine of the Spirit as it relates to the believer has over the last half-century been shrouded in a mist such as lies upon a mountain in stormy weather. A world of confusion has surrounded this truth. This confusion has not come by accident; an enemy has done this. Satan knows that Spiritless Evangelicalism is as deadly as modernism or heresy, and he has done everything in his power to prevent us from enjoying our true Christian heritage."

In Ephesians 5:18 we see four important truths on the filling of the Holy Spirit:

1. *It is commanded.* Ephesians 5:18 states, "Do not be drunk with wine, in which is dissipation, but be filled with the Spirit." We are commanded to be controlled by the Holy Spirit and not by alcohol or anything else in our lives. This filling and the control that results from it is not to be an option for us; the Greek verb for "be filled" indicates a command rather than an option. Failure to be filled by the Holy Spirit is disobedience and a sin.

2. *It is comprehensive.* The commandment to be filled literally addresses "you all" and refers to *each and every Christian*. *All* Christians are to be filled, not just missionaries or preachers. Charles Finney wrote, "He who neglects to obey the command to be filled with the Holy Spirit is as guilty of breaking the command of God as he who steals or curses or commits adultery. His guilt is as the authority of God is great, who commands us to be filled. His guilt is equivalent to all the good he might do if he were filled with the Spirit. " God will look at all the things a person

could have done had he been filled with the Holy Spirit, and will demand an accounting.

Trying to function as a Christian without the filling of the Holy Spirit is like trying to drive a car without enough oil in the engine. Oil is the lubricant that makes an engine run smoothly. An inadequate supply causes heat in the engine as it labors with friction and stress. Our spiritual engines experience a similar heat, felt as stress or anxiety, when we try to operate without the filling of the Holy Spirit. We become engines without oil.

3. *It is continual.* The continual-action verb "be filled" means literally "be being filled continually." The filling of the Holy Spirit must be *continual* lest our enemy find us lacking in God's power. Remember that lion roaming around seeking to destroy us? When Satan finds us filled to the brim with the Holy Spirit and possessing all the power that God has made available to us, Satan will not engage us in battle; he will wait for a more advantageous time. Satan wants nothing to do with us when we have bathed ourselves with God's Word and spent time in prayer, for then we are ready to do spiritual battle.

    Satan also knows when we are not continually being filled. As he prowls about, his eyes fall on a Christian whose life has a void in it due to the lack of the Holy Spirit. Without so much as an introduction, he moves in. We may be filled with the Spirit 30 days out of 31, and yet Satan will attack us on the one day when our engines are nearly empty of the oil of the Holy Spirit.

4. *It is controlling.* Recently Evander Holyfield and Riddick Bowe battled for the Heavyweight Boxing Championship of the world. Bowe won the bout in a decision. Before the bout each man put on gloves designed to soften the punches and protect his hands. Had I put Riddick Bowe's gloves on my hands, there would have been a different outcome to the fight! Although the gloves are important, it is the *hands inside* that generate the power.

There are other types of gloves which when worn by particular people will provide a garden of grandeur or build a beautiful piece of willow furniture. But take these gloves off and lay them aside, and they are worthless. *The power to create is not in the glove but in the hand inside it.*

We as Christians are like a pair of gloves. When we allow the Holy Spirit to reach in and fill our lives, He has the ability to create great works of art with them. Unfortunately, many Christians are like gloves sitting on the counter, waiting to be used someday.

THE SECRET OF STRENGTH

There are three main ingredients in experiencing a Spirit-filled life. The first is *our salvation.* To be saved we need to acknowledge that we are sinners incapable of paying the penalty for our own sins. Because of God's grace and love He sent His own Son to die for us. When Jesus was crucified, He paid sin's penalty once and for all. Then Jesus rose victorious from the grave, and by so doing conquered sin and death. Acts 16:31 tells us to "believe on the Lord Jesus Christ and you will be saved."

This belief is not just a casual acknowledgment that there is a God. It is a belief in *the finished work of the Savior dying and rising.* Have you asked Jesus to be your Savior? It is the most important step you can take in your life. There is a great struggle for our souls going on constantly as Satan and the Holy Spirit war over us. We experience the stress of these battles until we submit to God. The first step in outsmarting stress is to make peace with God and accept His sacrifice.

The second ingredient in the filling of the Holy Spirit is *our submission to Christ.* D. L. Moody used a glass of water to illustrate the power of submission. To stress his point he held up an empty glass and challenged the crowd to tell him how to get all the air out of the glass. One person said, "Suck it out with a pump," to which Moody replied, "That would create a vacuum and shatter the glass."

After several other impossible suggestions, Moody took a pitcher of water and simply poured it into the glass until it overflowed. Not a bit of air was left in the glass! Why? Because it became filled with water and there was no room left for air.

Victory in the Christian life comes not by "sucking out a sin here and there" but rather by *being filled with the Holy Spirit.* If we obey God, we will be so filled with the Holy Spirit that Satan will not be able to interfere in our lives and cause us to sin. Unfortunately, these glasses of ours have little cracks in them and seem to be constantly losing water. But there is a way to keep even a cracked glass filled: Just hold it directly under the spigot and let the water continually flow into it. The only way a Christian can be continually filled with God's Holy Spirit is to hold his life under the spigot of God daily and let God's power flow into it.

The third ingredient in the filling of the Holy Spirit is *our service to God.* If we are saved and submitted, serving should be a natural outgrowth in our lives. One of the best ways to serve God is by sharing Jesus with others. The reason many Christians fail to see the supernatural working of God's Holy Spirit is that they have never given Him a chance to "show His stuff." They live their lives cautiously, never taking a step of faith.

Sharing Jesus Christ with others means confronting people with their need of salvation. Perhaps it starts with an invitation to church or to our home for a neighborhood Bible study. Maybe it involves just being a friend. Many Christians do not challenge God to show His power, and so they never see Him at work. They fail to pray for legitimate things, and so they never see answers to their prayers.

Each of us has the potential to reach the special world that God has placed around us. Each person's influence is as different as the people in his particular world. These are the people who live next door or who work beside us; for some special reason God has placed them in our world. Perhaps God has been working in their hearts without our knowledge. He simply calls on us to share our lives with them and to tell them of what He has accomplished in our day-to-day struggles. We need to give God a chance to show what He can do. We don't need to save these people, since only God can do that, but we do need to tell them how He saved us and how He can save them too.

FRINGE BENEFITS

The Spirit-filled believer will be filled with the joy described in Ephesians 5:19-21: "Speaking to one another in songs and hymns and spiritual songs, singing and making melody in your heart to the Lord, giving thanks always for all things to God the Father in the name of our Lord Jesus Christ, submitting to one another in the fear of God."

Along with that joy comes great *power.* "You shall receive power when the Holy Spirit has come upon you, and you shall be witnesses to me in Jerusalem, and in all Judea and Samaria, and to the end of the earth" (Acts 1:8).

The Holy Spirit also gives *comfort*. In John 14:16-18 the writer says Jesus was about to ascend to heaven, but before He left He promised that He would send the Comforter, who is the Holy Spirit. He can comfort us because He knows us better than we know ourselves.

In addition, the Holy Spirit gives us *gifts* to help us serve God better. These gifts when properly used for God can bring unspeakable joy and fulfillment into our lives. He imparts *hope* in a world that has none to offer (John 14:17). He warns us of *wrongdoing* or *danger* (Hebrews 3:7-11). These are just a few of the fringe benefits which we receive along with the filling of the Holy Spirit.

As we look at all the unfolding events in the world around us, we can't help but think that Jesus is preparing to return soon, and we should rejoice in the thought. Yet some who call themselves Christians may actually fear His return. Are you one of these? Often people who were saved at a very young age, as I was, are not sure of their salvation. So let me challenge you to do something vitally important: *Don't finish reading this chapter until you are sure of your relationship with Christ.* One of the greatest qualities of the Holy Spirit is His ability to seal us forever with God. His loyalty and staying power are eternal.

The key to victorious Christian living is avoiding the control of our lives by anyone or anything other than the Holy Spirit. Satan will try to defile your life and make you doubt everything you know to be true of God and His character. To help you combat this vicious attack, God has promised you perfect peace and full assurance if you are willing to submit completely to Him.

4

....

STRESS-CONQUERING MARRIAGE

One of our recent Thanksgivings was undoubtedly the quietest our household has ever enjoyed. Due to a severe case of laryngitis, I was forced to sit around and listen while everybody else did the talking. (Actually, the family seemed to enjoy the change!)

Unfortunately, this Thanksgiving was not nearly so peaceful for a particular family in Oklahoma. As they sat down to enjoy their holiday meal, the newly married young man discovered that his young bride had failed to thaw the turkey completely. The poor bird was still frozen solid inside! That being more than he could handle, the young man flew into a rage while his wife ran for safety out the front door. He grabbed the partially frozen bird and went after her. As she attempted to drive away, he threw the turkey through the windshield, grabbed her, and threatened to assault her with the frozen bird. What a day of Thanksgiving!

SAFE HAVEN OR BATTLEGROUND?

During the year-end holiday season the average American gains a couple of interesting things. First, the average American gains anywhere from four to seven pounds! The second gain that people experience is an *increase in stress*. The typical American suffers more stress during the holidays than during any other time of the year. Among the reasons for this increase are busy schedules, shortage of funds, and poor diets.

Marriages, which should be safe havens from stress, also feel the weight of the increased holiday stress. With tempers and nerves already raw from other pressures, little irritations can explode into major hurts.

Psychology Today recently listed 43 occurrences in life which one study has shown to be the most stressful. When listed by order of severity, number one was the death of a spouse. It was given a stress rating of 100 points. Number two, with 73 points, was divorce. Marital separation was number three, receiving nearly the same number of stress points as divorce. Of the top ten stress inducers, *four were marriage-related.* In this chapter we will show God's plan to make your marriage stress-resistant by greatly limiting the total amount of stress flowing into your marriage.

Although some stress in marriage is inevitable, it need not be insurmountable. Our goal will be to identify unnecessary stress in marriage and then see what we can do to resist it.

HOT TUB INTRIGUE

God provided the basic guidelines for a healthy, happy marriage in Ephesians 5:22-29 when He declared, "Wives, submit to your own husbands, as to the Lord. For the husband is head of the wife, as Christ is head of the church; and He is the Savior of the body. Therefore, just as the church is subject to Christ, so let the wives be to their own husbands in everything. Husbands, love your wives, just as Christ also loved the church and gave Himself for it, that He might sanctify and cleanse it with the washing of water by the Word, that He might present it to Himself a glorious church, not having spot or wrinkle or any such thing, but that it should be holy and without blemish. So husbands ought to love their own wives as their own bodies; he who loves his wife loves himself. For no one ever hated his own flesh, but nourishes it and cherishes it, just as the Lord does the church."

If a husband and wife would adhere steadfastly to these principles, their marriage would be a refuge of joy. Unfortunately, these guidelines are often ignored. Let me describe a scene that could easily have happened near our church in Northern San Diego County.

It involves the attractive young wife of a U.S. Marine stationed at Camp Pendleton who has recently been deployed to the Mideast. His marriage was not strong prior to his departure, and this period of separation is likely to make or break their relationship. He is a career man who has always placed the Marine Corps ahead of everything else, including his wife.

Soon after his departure, his wife begins to experience a severe loneliness which seems to grow stronger with each passing day. One evening as she is lounging in the hot tub in the backyard, the attractive middle-aged executive who lives next door notices her. He has seen her before, but never like this.

Although considered successful by his friends, his marriage has long since lost its spark of joy. As his gaze lingers, he fantasizes how much happier he would be with his neighbor's wife. One thing leads to another, and soon they have become intimate with each other. Before long two marriages come crashing down.

ROOFTOP ROMANCE

Although this type of affair happens daily across our land, it is certainly not something which originated in the 1990s. Let me show you the same affair but with different faces as it occurred many years ago. Second Samuel 11:1-5 recounts the story.

"It came to pass in the spring of the year, at the time when kings go out to battle, that David sent Joab and his servants with him, and all Israel; and they destroyed the people of Ammon and besieged Rabbah, but David remained in Jerusalem. Then it happened one evening that David arose from his bed and walked on the roof of the king's house. And from the roof he saw a woman bathing, and the woman was very beautiful to behold. So David sent and inquired about the woman. And someone said, 'Is this not Bathsheba, the daughter of Eliam, the wife of Uriah the Hittite?' Then David sent messengers, and took her; and she came to him, and he lay with her, for she was cleansed from her impurity; and she returned to her house. And the woman conceived; so she sent and told David, and said, 'I am with child.'"

This story should have ended when David first saw Bathsheba bathing. He should have recognized the potential for disaster and continued his walk any place other than where he was. Instead, he chose to remain on the rooftop staring at the enticing beauty of another man's wife. He may have tried to justify his thoughts because of the loneliness he felt from his own marriage. But instead of fleeing, David put his feelings into action. In the passion of the moments which were to follow, he and Bathsheba would cause lives to be shattered and bring scars of guilt and stress that would last for the rest of their lives.

PAYING THE PRICE

Unbearable and yet unnecessary stress can infiltrate the strongest of marriages during a single unguarded moment. Because the cost of carelessness in relationships is so painful, we must be constantly aware of our feelings and intentions, and guard them carefully. There is no stress quite as severe as that which accompanies the breach of the marriage vows.

David could not escape the cost of the sin spreading through his life like a cancer. Because of David's special relationship with God he agonized over his sins and sought God's forgiveness. David's greatest hurt was over the loss of precious fellowship with God. Although he was forgiven by God, the scars remained to haunt him the rest of his days. David and Bathsheba's baby died shortly after birth. His wives were publicly violated. His family suffered the shame of rebellion, rape, and murder. The kingdom that God had given him was never at peace. Even though David was known for his many military victories, to this day marital infidelity by Christian leaders is still referred to as "David's sin."

ADVERTISING FOR DISASTER

After reading and rereading the account of David and Bathsheba, I am convinced that there were no innocent victims in their affair. This is consistent with my experience in marriage counseling. In nearly every situation, the finger of fault points in some degree to all of the people involved.

In trying to understand what contributed to the downfall of these two marriages, I don't get the picture of Bathsheba as an innocent and helpless woman who was victimized by a ruthless king. We must remember that she was naked and bathing while in clear view of the king's balcony. She knew exactly what she was doing and perhaps wanted to be seen. Due to the absence of her husband, her marriage may already have been weak, and her actions served to further undermine it. At the very least her behavior was quite provocative. Such behavior is one of several ways that married men or women may be advertising for disaster. Here are some behaviors which can cause the foundation of a marriage to crumble.

PROVOCATIVE DRESS

Although styles change, decency remains constant. Each generation has a fairly clear consensus of what is or isn't considered modest. I went to college during the days of the miniskirt, and oh, what arguments raged between girls and their parents over the length of skirts!

It is important to remember that not all miniskirts were created equal. Some were accepted as decent while others pushed the concept of "short" to the point that they were considered provocative. Despite ever-changing fashions, people have a socially accepted standard which allows them to know when someone is advertising for the wrong kind of attention. But even in our so called "sexually liberated" society, splashing around nude in full view of the public would be considered provocative behavior.

FLIRTATIOUS BEHAVIOR

A second way to advertise for disaster is through flirtatious behavior. Unfortunately, some people never stop seeking attention from members of the opposite sex even after they are married. Such flirtatious behavior can do grave harm to a marriage. Manifesting itself in numerous ways, it may simply be the manner in which an individual talks with members of the opposite sex. He (or she) may enjoy bringing up intimate topics even though he claims he is "only kidding."

Flirtatious behavior may also involve those "friendly" kisses and hugs shared with close friends of the family. There are several kinds of hugs; some are innocent tokens of true friendship while others are intended by the "hugger" to arouse desire in the heart of the "huggee."

If you experience the desire to hug the spouse of another person for the wrong reason, better not to hug at all. You never know how the person at the other end of the hug might respond to what he or she interprets as flirtatious behavior. Satan has an uncanny way of putting people in just the "wrong" situations at just the "right" times.

EXPLOSIVE SITUATIONS

A person may also be advertising for disaster by allowing himself to get caught in explosive situations. These almost always involve circumstances in which members of the opposite sex are alone with each other.

One of the safest ways to maintain personal fidelity is to flee situations that could get out of hand. Unfortunately, once our hormones kick into gear it is very difficult for our brain to apply the brakes. Many an affair began innocently enough but soon ripened to a level that the couple couldn't control. The Holy Spirit is quite capable of warning us as we approach such dangerous situations; the problem is that we usually know exactly what we're doing but aren't willing to respond to His voice.

KEEP THE HOME FIRES HOT

It never fails to amaze me how much external stress a couple can endure when their personal relationship is strong. Seldom are partners tempted to wander when there is contentment at home. There is no need or desire to seek warmth around another fire when there is adequate warmth at home. It is *when the home fire has died down and grown cold* that couples become vulnerable to all sorts of temptations.

David sought the warmth of another man's fire in his relationship with Bathsheba. As a result of the affair and the pregnancy that resulted, David felt the shame and stress of having to try to cover his tracks. Everybody knew that Uriah was off to war and could not have fathered the child. How would Bathsheba explain her pregnancy? Justice might demand that she be stoned to death for her adultery.

Hoping to remedy the problem, David fabricated an excuse to have Uriah return to Jerusalem. David was convinced that while home, Uriah would lie with his wife and believe the child was his own.

The first phase of the plan worked smoothly as Uriah was called back to Jerusalem to deliver a report to his commander-in-chief. But to King David's dismay, on two separate occasions Uriah refused to go in to his wife.

Although much has been made of David's conniving and sin in this affair, let the finger of fault not overlook Uriah and his mistreatment of his young wife. She certainly had cause to question his love. Although this does not excuse her sin, it does help us to understand its foundation. Uriah may have been a good soldier, but as a husband he was sadly deficient. Uriah's problems may have developed because he placed his career ahead of his wife.

IT STARTS WITH THE MAN

In the numerous cases of marital conflict with which I have dealt, it is almost always the husband who is initially at fault.

Many are the times I have answered the telephone only to discover on the other end of the line a desperate man who has just learned that his wife wants out of the marriage. He acts truly shocked at her apparent unfaithfulness, and wants me to explain to him what is wrong with her. As we then begin to trace their history, years and sometimes decades, of neglect and abuse of the wife by the husband are brought to the surface.

As a rule, women are remarkably devoted to their men. They walk out of the wedding ceremony humming the tune "Stand by Your Man" and mean to do just that until death do them part. Normally, it takes a tremendous amount of abuse, neglect, or coldness before a wife finally walks away from a marriage. Unfortunately, when she reaches the point where she has had enough she means it, and under most circumstances will not be deterred from leaving. I have enjoyed only limited success in salvaging marriages which have reached this stage.

How can we keep the home fires hot and cause love to continue to grow? How can we rekindle a marriage that has already cooled off? Here are some principles which can earn you straight A's in your marriage.

NOTICE YOUR SPOUSE

You can begin by noticing your spouse and giving him or her the attention he or she needs and deserves. Believe me, if you don't, someone else will! Perhaps other people don't see the unkempt beard or the rollers you see daily, or gaze into the weary eyes of the parent who has been up all night with a sick child. All they see is the handsome executive or the lovely secretary who is always at his or her best at work.

Many times spouses need encouragement to keep up their appearance while at home. Daily mundane chores and responsibilities may distract them from this important part of their relationship. You can accomplish much more by encouragement than by criticism.

Perhaps your wife has just bought a new dress. Even though you may not love the dress, your wife does. You ought to be the first to compliment her rather than complain about how much it cost or be critical of how it looks on her. Because of your simple act of showing attention, next time she may ask for your help in choosing a dress. This is the time to express your preference. Remember, it is *the person inside the dress* whom you love, and not what she is wearing.

Wives, when your husband works hard getting in shape or accomplishing a goal he has been striving for, shower him with praise and encourage him to keep up the good work. You need to let him know that he's looking good and that you appreciate the hard work it takes to keep in shape.

Attention begins by verbally assuring your spouse that you love him or her. Even though he may know that you love him, he will thrive on being repeatedly reminded of it.

We live in a world that tries to sell love cheaply. People no longer look at marriage as something for keeps; it has become just as disposable as everything else. A strong Christian marriage is a living miracle these days. The home where Mom and Dad are secure in their love for each other and where the children can go to bed confident that Mom and Dad are deeply in love has become a rarity in our society. Children grow more secure as they daily witness the attention their parents show each other.

Couples face many struggles as they try to keep their marriages alive and well. One of the most difficult struggles my wife and I face is finding time together without five loving children either hanging onto us for attention or wanting to be taken to this or that place. Although we love our children and enjoy their company, we know that our marriage can't be built around them alone.

Many outwardly successful marriages seem to disintegrate when the kids finally leave home, even though up until that time everything appeared fine. Life is a bustle of activity as Mom and Dad spend their evenings and weekends chauffeuring children to assorted lessons, practices, and friends' homes. It's the typical American family, and as in other families the day eventually arrives when the last child leaves the nest and it's just Mom and Dad alone again. Mom stares across the dining room table at a man who seems like a virtual stranger. They have spent years giving attention to everybody but each other, only to discover now that the person who has made such a wonderful parent is not such a wonderful spouse.

BACK TO MEMORY LANE

Let's do a little walking down memory lane. Take a minute to think back to the time when you fell in love. Remember the excitement of those days? Have you ever tried to figure out why you fell in love with that particular person? The key probably had a lot to do with *romance* or *affection*.

In those early days and months of romance, flowers and gifts were frequently given. An evening couldn't slip by without spending at least a half-hour together on the telephone. Dates took place at least two or three times a week. Much time was spent making sure that hair and clothes were always in perfect condition. Finally—after the candy, flowers, careful caring for appearance, and many letters and phone calls—came marriage.

Not long after the thrill of the wedding had subsided, "dates" became a thing of the past as you both had jobs and worked overtime to pay for the house, two cars, furniture, and before long, the children. With luck, perhaps you had Saturdays together, but by then you were so worn out that you didn't care if you shaved, put on makeup, or did anything to show concern for your appearance. When asked why, you might have responded, "Well, I'm not planning on seeing anyone important today." As far as spending meaningful time together, the majority of your free time was spent in front of the TV watching the Simpsons or Monday Night Football. Then you crawled up to bed and mumbled good night to each other . . . and goodbye to romance. You still loved each other, but with each passing year the romance and affection became a fainter memory.

King David had a wife named Abigail. She was the one in hair curlers and tattered bathrobe caring for the sick kids and dirty dishes. Like husbands since the beginning of time, David saw his wife at her worst each morning.

This happens daily across America. Husbands kiss wives who have spent their morning dressing and feeding kids to send them off to school good-bye. As on so many other mornings, they couldn't get the kids up on time, no one liked the cereal that was left, and besides there was no more milk anyway. Dad's shirt wasn't ironed yet, and he forgot to tell her that he had to be in the office early, so she'll have to drive the kids to school. She can just throw on something because she won't be seeing anyone important anyway. Instead of a warm "Have a nice day today, honey" he receives a tongue-lashing because he forgot to fix the garbage disposal the night before, and there's a sink load of dishes from the last two days waiting to be washed.

Many are the men and women who head for work with their insides rumbling from the stress of a hurried morning.

Jobs often become welcome havens from the storms at home. Some men arrive at the office vulnerable to the enticements that await them.

LEARN TO ACCEPT

Premarital counseling never fails to fascinate me. Although the young couples I counsel have never been married before, they feel they know everything there is to know about marriage. They have the whole program figured out.

Many times as the sessions unearth areas of potential concern, my attempts to address these are rebuffed with the idea that he or she will change for the better after they are married. In reality, however, the chances of such change are slim when it comes to a spouse. If you are thinking of marrying a person with some undesirable characteristics, remember that these problems are likely to get *worse* rather than better after the wedding.

This is especially true of men with explosive tempers. His bride-to-be is convinced that she will be able to break him of this dangerous problem once they are wed. Unfortunately, she is wrong, and is more likely to end up with a frozen turkey tossed through her windshield one day in the future. The secret is to find someone who is acceptable "as is." If there is something about him (or her) which you can't tolerate now, don't marry him. Make these decisions before you become so blinded by love that you can't think clearly.

For those who are already married to a person who is less than perfect (and that includes all of us), we need to learn the art of *acceptance*. Although one's spouse may lack some of the strengths of another person, accept him or her for his strengths. Often we spend so much time criticizing weaknesses that we destroy the strengths at the same time. Many men expect their wives to be perfect, and make them feel guilty for falling short of this lofty and unrealistic standard. They are critical of their wives because they want them to look like Cindy Crawford and cook like Betty Crocker.

Many a devoted wife has not only borne children but also the stress of nurturing and feeding and providing for their emotional and physical needs. Many times this occurs at the expense of their own health and spare time. They may not cook like Betty Crocker, but they sure know by memory the cookbook on Fixing Chicken and Hamburger 1000 Ways! They can run the household with incredible accountability, knowing the hiding place of every sock and mislaid article. I have a feeling that the successful housewife could run just about any large corporation, since she has on-the-job experience in all levels of management.

Wives have the tendency to compare their husbands with those of their friends. It frustrates her that he doesn't have her drive and desire for bigger and better things. He's just a happy-go-lucky guy who lets the cares of the world roll off his shoulders. He may be a very romantic person who loves to do special things for her, but all she thinks about is how much this and that costs. Why can't he just be more like so and so!

A wife needs to learn to accept her spouse for who he is. Her husband may not be the most driven man in the world, but he is blessed with a mellow personality that allows him to come home and enjoy his family regardless of what the world has dumped on him that day. He knows how to roll with the punches and not stress out his family with his problems. He may be man enough to acknowledge that his wife is a better money manager than he is, and is therefore comfortable in letting her exercise her gift. (To other men this would be very threatening.)

There are many women who would trade anything for a husband who knows how to be romantic and would think to give them a gift. Don't make the mistake of continually comparing *your* spouse to someone else's spouse. Let him know that you accept and love him for who he is.

SHOW YOUR APPRECIATION

I've known a number of men who, through God's kindness, married far better than they deserved. Their success in life is largely a result of the efforts of their wife. She is the one who has organized and implemented his work. In many cases she is the one who has brought up their children in the nurture and admonition of the Lord in periods of his absence. All men in general and these men in particular should have the wisdom to express their appreciation generously.

Many times men receive appreciation and gratification on the job through raises and promotions, but rarely does a mother or wife get a raise or a promotion. My wife was feeling the need for such a raise or promotion several years ago. Although she was happily raising our children and busily working within our church ministries, she felt a sense of loss in her life. The fruits of labor for the typical mother and wife aren't as evident as they should be. I assured her that my accomplishments were hers also, and that without her being there to care for the needs of the family in her own special way, I would not have the freedom to do what God had called me to do. She understood and agreed, but she still needed to hear that what she was doing did make a difference. That's why I dedicated this book to Carolyn.

Men need to be creative in the ways they demonstrate their thanks and appreciation for what their wives do, and they need to teach their children to do the same. This is especially true of those wives who not only manage the household but also hold a job outside the home. In addition to verbal appreciation, they need the whole family's support in caring for the house.

Likewise, wives need to show their husbands appreciation for all they do for them and the children. By observation the children will learn that appreciation is one of the most valuable gifts that can be given to their father. He may not do everything perfectly, but when he does what he can, his family needs to be quick to let him know that it is noticed and appreciated. If we have two parents who practice appreciation in their relationship, their children will very likely practice it also.

LOOKING GOOD WHERE IT COUNTS

As you prepare yourselves for the day have you ever considered who it is that you are trying to impress with your appearance? We ought not to leave the house thinking about how good we will look for others until we have first tried to look our best for our own families. They are the most important people we will see, so let's make sure to look good for them first.

Although it's true that looks aren't everything, appearance can have a positive or a negative influence on a marriage. Physical attractiveness can add sizzle and stave off a wandering eye in a marriage. Each partner should strive to maintain a pleasing appearance for his or her spouse.

IS YOUR ARMOR ON?

David was accustomed to putting on his armor before battle. He knew of his need for protection from those mortal blows from the enemy. Where he grew careless was in not arming himself against a much greater enemy than those who fought against Israel. Satan was and is a formidable enemy; his blows are usually underhanded and unexpected. David was vulnerable one evening and went out unprepared to resist Satan's weapon called temptation.

The scene is set in 2 Samuel 11:1, "It came to pass in the spring of the year, at the time when kings go out to battle." Wait a minute! If David is king, shouldn't he be leading his army in battle? It's spring, and his armies are off to battle. David *sent* them but chose not to *lead* them. Instead, he was back in Jerusalem wrestling with a restless spirit. He no doubt walked often in the evening around the palace walls, perhaps thinking about how his armies were doing. But instead of putting his spirit to rest by joining up with his armies, he became distracted by Bathsheba. Because David was not busy doing his assigned work for God, a vacuum was created. Vacuums do not occur naturally in nature, and are always quickly filled. Needless to say, it didn't take Satan long to fill the vacuum in David's life.

David probably never thought he would face the battle of his life in his own backyard, but Satan has a keen sense of timing. He can put just the right temptation in a person's life at just the right moment, and even help a person justify it in his mind. It is to Satan's advantage to use the element of surprise in his attacks. Our only defense is a good offense: *If we want war we need only prepare for peace, but if we want true personal peace we must constantly prepare for war!*

5
....

MARITAL MINEFIELDS

Marriage is a serious business. It involves the signing of a legally binding contract by a pair of young adults who are so madly in love with each other that they are absolutely blind to the realities of life. While in this vulnerable condition, they enter into a lifetime contract which they vow to honor until death parts them.

Soon thereafter, as stress begins to build, these same two people are ready to do anything possible to get out of this contract . . . sometimes even killing each other to do it. They imagine that by escaping their marital bond and the responsibilities that come with it, the stresses they are feeling will somehow go away. As they find themselves fighting in court over this or that, what started out as a declaration of *love* has turned into a declaration of *war*.

Ephesians 5:30-33 states, "We are members of His body, of His flesh and of His bones. For this reason a man shall leave his father and mother and be joined to his wife, and the two shall become one flesh. This is a great mystery, but I speak concerning Christ and the church. Nevertheless let each one of you in particular so love his own wife as himself, and let the wife see that she respects her husband." In referring to His relationship with the church Christ used the words "a great mystery" to explain its complexity.

A similar "great mystery" exists in the marriage relationship of a man and a woman. Marriage is the blending of two separate worlds into one. When it works well, it is truly a miracle to behold. When it fails, it is of all things most miserable to endure.

STRIFE FROM VARIETY?

Each of the partners entering into a marriage contract has been raised differently from his or her new spouse. They may have been raised in a home with their two biological parents, or a single parent, or a stepparent, or possibly in a home with neither of their parents. They may have grown up alone or surrounded by one or many brothers or sisters. Perhaps their parents were well off financially, or possibly they struggled constantly just to make ends meet. One partner may have been raised with little or no discipline while the other lived with overbearing discipline. Perhaps one home had an abusive parent or brother or sister. Added to this is the unique personality given to each person at conception which has been either nurtured or suppressed under all the previous conditions.

Some of these differences can bring wonderful change and growth in marriage. Others may drive a wedge between the parties involved that can literally start all-out war. We joke about couples who fight over how to roll up a toothpaste tube or who will take out the garbage, but such frustrations can add the last straw to an already fragile relationship. Raising children, paying mounting bills, coping with poor health, and struggling with an oppressing job, when added to an already-complex relationship, can send a couple over the edge if they are not functioning as a united team.

Of the many obstacles that married couples face, the ones that are avoidable are sometimes the most dangerous. Many times we cannot control long-term illness or the loss of a job that robs us of the ability to pay our bills. But what we do have control over is our response to the circumstances we face, and whether we will let these bond us together like glue or blow us apart.

MAPPING THE MINEFIELDS

In times of war, armies bury landmines under the earth in areas known as minefields. When their unsuspecting enemy wanders into these fields, they are likely to step on one or more mines and trigger explosions. If the soldiers are aware of where these minefields are located, they can spare themselves great pain and loss by simply avoiding them.

As Christians we have an adversary who roams around seeking ways to destroy our marriages. Our enemy's name is Satan, and by his design our lives are surrounded by hidden minefields. One step in the wrong direction can bring destruction not only to us but also to those close to us. To protect our marriages, God warns us in His Word to avoid Satan's land mines by keeping watch over our thoughts, words, and actions. We are to focus our attention on our spouse and families. When distracted from them by others we can find ourselves lost and alone in a marital minefield.

Here are some common types of land mines that Satan uses to cause strife in the marriage of a careless Christian.

ALONE IN THE DANGER ZONE

Disaster can occur when a married man or woman is alone with a member of the opposite sex other than his or her spouse. King David certainly found this to be true. Although he was headed for trouble as he watched Bathsheba bathe, disaster struck when he sent for her and they spent time together. When he purposely chose to see her alone, being fully aware of the lust burning in his heart, his fate was sealed. There would be no turning back once David was alone with Bathsheba.

Sometimes we find ourselves alone with the spouse of another person without our choosing. Once as my wife and I were about to leave the house to meet another couple for a relaxing dinner, I made the mistake of answering the phone as we went out the front door. The caller was obviously distraught as he blurted out, "My wife and I need to see you immediately. I'm afraid she's about to leave me." I asked if I could come by after dinner, but he was convinced that every wasted moment could be the last for their marriage.

Reluctantly we canceled our dinner date and I headed over to meet him at his house. Upon arrival I discovered a wife with no knowledge of where her husband was. This left me sitting in another man's home, situated down a secluded road, alone with his wife. After making small talk for more than an hour I felt it would be prudent for me to leave. I left my phone number in case the "emergency" resurrected.

I never received a phone call back from the distraught husband, and the next time I saw him he said nothing about the incident. I finally pulled him aside and asked for an explanation. He just laughed and explained that right after he hung up he remembered a potential client he wanted to see and decided to stop by on his way home. It turned out his client was ready to buy, and so he spent several hours drawing up a very lucrative sale.

I felt as if I had been tricked into the middle of a minefield and then left there. Although I didn't expect or choose to be in such a situation, the danger was just as real as if I had. One careless move on my part while down that secluded road, and my whole ministry could have exploded into ruin. Fortunately, I survived this potential minefield because I recognized the danger and fled.

INTRIGUE AT THE OFFICE

The office or workplace can likewise prove to be an extremely dangerous minefield. Relationships can develop quite innocently when people work together. They can develop a strong camaraderie when they join forces to tackle challenges as well as frustrations on a daily basis.

They never see each other except when they are at their best. She may marvel at how he always takes charge of a situation and never criticizes her—she gets enough of that at home. Meanwhile he is amazed that his secretary always looks beautiful and is so well organized. She really seems to have her act together. (At home things are always a mess, and he can never find anything.) He may begin to wish his wife could look and act more like his secretary. If the truth were known, he may have chosen to hire her in the first place because she represented what he was looking for in the perfect woman. They now find themselves daily walking through a minefield.

The relationships formed at work are important. They make our jobs more enjoyable and we can learn a great deal from each other. But because of the unusual working arrangements that occur, such as late hours, business trips, etc., there will always be occasion for stepping out of line with one another. Realizing the potential for these problems, God warns us in Ephesians 5:22 to show great caution: "Wives, submit to your own husbands." This does not mean that women can never work for men other than their husbands, but that they must be very careful about the relationships they make while at work. The same applies to men.

The verse also implies that men who have married women working for them need to be careful of their expectations from them. When a married man or woman looks to his or her employer or employee for anything other than a hard day's work, he is disobeying God's Word and opening himself up for disaster.

GUEST OF PERIL

Another potential minefield awaits us in the area of overnight or frequent hospitality. We've all experienced situations where a houseguest wound up staying longer than we expected or was wise, or came over more often than he or she should. If the houseguest is either single or away from his spouse, we need to take extra care to avoid being alone with him if he is of the opposite sex. People who normally wouldn't attract our attention often become desirable to us as we grow more comfortable with them.

I have worked with a number of couples in which one of the partners has accused the other of having an affair with their houseguest. Each time I've sat down with them in my office and asked the accused whether anything has been or currently is going on, I have been told with indignation that he or she is absolutely innocent of any wrongdoing. Time tells all, and eventually I discover that there was an affair after all.

We can be hospitable to our world around us and freely open our homes to others, but we need to be extra careful when entertaining others to keep our hospitality something that is truly God-honoring, with our only motive being to show His love.

THE COUNSELING MINEFIELD

Whenever you begin to counsel a member of the opposite sex, you enter a loaded minefield. Although this should not prevent you from sharing advice with friends who seek it, you must be aware of the potential for great damage. Problems can develop when the same person continually seeks your help and pours out his or her problems to you instead of allowing someone of his own sex to guide him through his difficulties.

One of the most common causes of marital dysfunction occurs when husbands refuse to talk or listen to their wives. With this as a backdrop, the lonely and frustrated wife finally discovers a man who will listen to her and express true concern about her feelings. It doesn't take many counseling sessions for a strong bond to be forged between the two.

Knowing our nature and our tendency to be drawn toward members of the opposite sex, God has made it clear who should counsel the younger women. Titus 2:2-5 exhorts, "The older women likewise, that they be reverent in behavior, not slanderers, not given to much wine, teachers of all things—that they admonish the young women to love their husbands, to love their children, to be discreet, chaste, homemakers, good, obedient to their own husbands, that the word of God may not be blasphemed." If older women in churches would obey this instruction, fewer pastors would fall into the sin of infidelity!

But men are not the only ones who face danger in the "counseling minefield." Sometimes sympathizing women wind up counseling and consoling lonely men who pour out all their innermost hurts and needs. These men have lost communication with their wives and feel more comfortable talking things out with a woman than with their own male friends. As the two share their deepest feelings and frustrations, they are drawn closer to each other than to their spouses. Now all they need for disaster to strike is one unguarded moment.

Other women have been caught in the trap of hoping they can win a male friend to Christ by witnessing to him. Some men use this desire to keep the woman at hand, never intending to actually accept Christ. The best solution to this dilemma is to turn him over to a husband or other male friend to continue the counseling. If his heart is truly open to God, the Holy Spirit can complete His work much more effectively without a woman as a distraction.

RUSHING FOR THE FAST TRACK

A wise old preacher gave my wife and me some valuable premarital counsel when he suggested that we would greatly strengthen our relationship if in the early years of our marriage we would invest more in shared experiences than in shared possessions. We took his advice to heart and had some great vacations in our bright red VW Bug as we crossed the country from Plymouth Rock to Yellowstone National Park. We didn't have a lot of money to spend but we have great memories of those times because we were less encumbered with other responsibilities than we have been at any time since then.

This doesn't mean that we haven't suffered occasional cases of the "wants" for possessions we will probably never get. We simply have to make choices in these areas. Some choices are determined by our income while others are decided by our family size and lifestyle.

One big danger that many young couples face is trying to jump immediately onto the fast track of life. They want to complete college and graduate school, buy a new house and all the furnishings, and drive two new cars. They want today what their parents worked 30 years to acquire. Because the two of them hold jobs with conflicting hours and lots of overtime, they are not able to spend much time together, but they are at least able to stay current on all their bills and charge cards. But then one evening the wife reports that she is expecting. They are excited about this new development but wonder how in the world they will survive financially, since they have become slaves to large monthly payments. (Sometimes couples wrestle with the repercussions of their early spending habits for decades to come.)

Now the wife discovers that she can no longer work due to the pregnancy. In response, her husband determines to drop out of college and look for a job that will help cover the loss of her income. Many times neither of them is ever able to complete his or her education, so they spend their lives working at a job they never really wanted to hold. Then they suffer the lack of fulfillment of dreams and goals.

SPOTS IN THE GREEN GRASS

Twenty years have now passed since our young couple first married. Their children are almost grown, and Dad is finally trying to finish college, since the past two decades have been one struggle after another. Dad was unable to get a better job because he lacked the proper qualifications, and Mom has been out of the job market long enough to have obsolete job skills. Although they have enjoyed raising their children, they have drifted apart in their marital relationship, since everything in their lives for the last two decades has been child-centered.

They have now reached a stage when many couples start to feel the losses in their lives. They look back, only to see dreams never reached and goals never attained. They look enviously at their friends and contemporaries who have apparently attained success in life and are happily reaping its fruit.

Mid-life can be a very difficult time for married couples; unique stresses bombard them from all directions. Their bodies are definitely changing, and they have gray hair and wrinkles to prove it. The world they grew up in, with its music and life-style, has been replaced by a strange and ever-changing world.

Those of us who are considered Baby Boomers can really identify with this phenomenon. We were raised in very affluent times, and our parents had great hopes for us. They wanted us to possess and experience all the things they never had.

Unfortunately, what resulted was a generation of kids who could never get enough and didn't really want what they got. They wanted to speak their own mind but didn't want to take the responsibility for what they said or did. We are a generation always looking at the greener grass on the other side of the hill.

I work hard to keep the grass in my yard looking if not good, at least respectable. After inspecting all the holes, weeds, and brown spots in my lawn, I marveled at my neighbor's lawn: It was the picture of green perfection, with hardly a weed to be seen.

Then one day I strolled across the street and happened to inspect his lawn up close and personal. Two facts were instantly brought to my attention: 1) His lawn was riddled with holes, weeds, and brown spots to a degree at least equal to mine, and 2) from his side of the street my lawn looked better than his! I had just encountered the myth of the greener grass.

Depending on the perspective or angle, things can appear to be either better or worse than they actually are. When standing real close we see only the imperfections and are likely to miss what beauty there may be. If, on the other hand, we view the same item from afar, we are likely to focus on its beauty while overlooking the ugly brown spots.

This same phenomenon can occur when observing people who are close to us as well as those who are distant from us. We tend to see the ugly brown spots in those who are close to us, while we see beauty in those at a distance. If we're not careful, we can enter a dangerous minefield because of this misperception.

David and Bathsheba's story is living proof of this danger. In his mid-life years, David had grown weary in his position as Commander of the forces of Israel. He and Abigail had been married for some time, enduring periods of long separation from each other. Their worlds had developed in two different directions, undermining the foundation of their marriage. Instead of seeking to remedy this situation, David looked over the fence at what he thought was a greener pasture. Perhaps he thought it would be so much easier and less stressful just to start all over. Abigail's weaknesses were so glaring while Bathsheba's beauties were so inviting.

However, once he was on the other side of the fence, it probably didn't take long for David to realize that Bathsheba also had a few weeds to pull. Also, I wonder what type of man Bathsheba thought David was as he planned her husband's death on the battlefield! Neither Bathsheba nor David realized the potholes they would find or the dirt they would have to shovel to fill them. Their vision of greener grass was just an illusion; what they were getting into was just a minefield in disguise.

No Clean Breaks

The people of my church know the majority of my strengths and weaknesses, as well as my likes and dislikes. They even know that I enjoy watching professional wrestling! Of course I know it's fake. As a matter of fact, the more outrageous the better.

At these matches you seldom see a "clean break" when the two entangled wrestlers are asked by the referee to separate. One of the two will invariably take a cheap shot at the other as they separate. There are few clean breaks in professional wrestling.

Neither are there clean breaks when the earth begins to shift. As we prepared to move to California from Michigan, we wondered how long it would be before we experienced our first earthquake. We didn't have to wait long . . . one occurred seven days after our arrival! As the faults underneath California break loose and rub against each other, they send the residents running for cover or out into the open spaces for safety. There are no clean breaks with earthquakes.

Marriages experience the same kind of rumblings when partners consistently rub each other the wrong way. Sometimes these marriages have lasted for as long as 40 years—or as little as 40 days. Without warning one of the two may file for divorce, and the long, arduous process of inflicting blame and pain begins.

California has what is called "no-fault divorce." They probably should have chosen another expression to describe it, because by the time a couple gets to court their marriage is so riddled with faults that quaking in the relationship is inevitable. Unfortunately, they have not yet come up with "no-pain divorce."

As families experience divorce, people feel its tremors all the way down the fault line. The children are nearly rattled to death as the parents fight over custody and finances. Generations down the family line feel the shaking long after "the Big One" hits. There is no such thing as a clean break when it comes to marriage.

If people could contemplate with the advantage of hindsight

the results of their actions, there would be far fewer shattered homes. Unfortunately, we don't have that advantage when we enter into a relationship outside of marriage. Knowing that it is both dangerous and wrong and yet burdened with loneliness, wants, bitterness, and a totally wrong perspective, we capriciously charge ahead, hoping that somehow no one will get hurt. We just want a clean break so we can start all over.

SHADOWED BY THE PAST

David and Bathsheba thought they had taken care of all the details when they forged ahead with their illicit relationship. Complicating the matter was the child who was to be born. After David removed Uriah from the picture he tried to convince himself that he had achieved a "clean break."

Second Samuel 12:1–12 provides the finishing touches to the story of David and Bathsheba.

> Then the Lord sent Nathan to David. And he came to him, and said to him: "There were two men in one city one rich and the other poor. The rich man had exceedingly many flocks and herds. But the poor man had nothing except one little ewe lamb which he had bought and nourished; and it grew up together with him and with his children. It ate of his own food and drank from his own cup and lay in his bosom; and it was like a daughter to him. And a traveler came to the rich man, who refused to take from his own flock and from his own herd to prepare one for the wayfaring man who had come to him; but he took the poor man's lamb and prepared it for the man who had come to him."
>
> Then David's anger was greatly aroused against the man, and he said to Nathan, "As the Lord lives, the man who has done this shall surely die! And he shall restore fourfold for the lamb, because he did this thing and because he had no pity."
>
> Then Nathan said to David, "You are the man! Thus says the Lord God of Israel: 'I anointed you king over Israel, and I delivered you from the hand of Saul. I gave you your master's house and your master's wives into your keeping, and gave you the house of Israel and Judah. And if that had been too little, I also would have given you much more! Why have you despised the commandment of the Lord, to do evil in His sight? You have killed Uriah the Hittite with the sword; you have taken his wife to be your wife, and have killed him with the sword of the people of Ammon. Now therefore, the sword shall never depart

from your house, because you have despised Me, and have taken the wife of Uriah the Hittite to be your wife.'

Thus says the Lord, 'Behold, I will raise up adversity against you from your own house; and I will take your wives before your eyes and give them to your neighbor, and he shall lie with your wives in the sight of this sun. For you did it secretly, but I will do this thing before all Israel, before the sun.'"

So much for the myth of the clean break! There was a whole lot of shaking and quaking going on in David's life and in the lives of his entire family because of his actions. His future plans for a happy life with Bathsheba were to be shadowed by God's condemnation of what he had done.

Many important lessons are available for each of us if we will be wise enough to learn from the mistakes of others.

First, we learn that there are never any secret sins. Because we sin against a God who sees and knows all things, just the knowledge of His watchful eye over us should keep us pure in thought, in word, and in deed. God tells us that if we lust after someone we are committing the sin of adultery in our minds. It might only be a matter of time before the thought is converted into action.

Second, we can be sure our sins will find us out. It is a very old saying, but so true yet today, that the sin of desire is referred to as a hot burning coal that will consume all those who attempt to hide it in their hearts. It will eventually burn its way to the surface of the man or woman who harbors it.

Third, we have no idea what we will miss in God's plan for our lives if we involve ourselves in sins that are evil in His sight. God told David that He would have given him what he desired if he had not despised His commandment. David not only lost what he had, but also what God was going to give him and allow him to do. David's dream was to build a temple in which God could dwell, but God took this honor from him and gave it to his son Solomon. David was left to lament that he alone had destroyed the most important of things—his ability to fulfill God's chosen will for his life.

SEDUCTION OF THE MIND

All sexual involvement outside of marriage is forbidden by God. This ought to be sufficient to settle this issue once and for all for every believer. As one old preacher used to say, "Just do what is right until the stars fall out of the sky." When we knowingly disobey God and choose to do wrong, we cause ourselves to undergo a stress that can destroy us both emotionally and physically. We can't possibly feel good about ourselves. The guilt that comes from violating our own bodies is multiplied by the breach of trust of our parents and those who look to us as an example. There is enough to think about during the days leading up to the wedding without complicating it with the shame and fear of pregnancy.

Regardless of a head knowledge of what is right, some couples find it more difficult to refrain from premarital sex after they have become engaged and the wedding date draws closer. They're getting married anyway, so why wait?

Studies show that couples engaged in sex prior to marriage double their chances of later having a relationship outside their marriage. The first violation is always the most difficult, and they have already put that one behind them. It now becomes easier to continue the pattern learned prior to marriage; they have already violated the sanctity of the marriage bond.

Many times in counseling situations, the wife declares her frustration with a husband who no longer exhibits interest in sex. She just can't understand it, because before they were married he was forever pressuring her for it. Finally, out of fear of losing the relationship, she gave in to him and lost her virginity. Although she didn't lose him at that time, it seems she has lost him now. What went wrong? It is my observation that one of the surest ways to end up with a passive husband with no interest in sex after marriage is to give him all he wants prior to marriage.

There are many culprits fighting for the seduction of the minds of men, women, and children today. Into our own homes, with the easy availability of television and movies, can come clear messages belittling the sanctity of marriage and the encouragement of sexual involvement without even the thought of marriage.

Much of modern entertainment is designed to sexually excite the viewer. If sex is predominant in a person's mind, he or she needs to examine his daily walk to see what kind of input he is receiving.

Many men have developed a false view of what their wife should be like because of the trash they are watching on TV.

They expect *sexual performance* instead of *true godly love.* They may feel defrauded because they are not experiencing at home the raw passion they are seeing on the screen. Pornography, whether hard-core or soft-core, will do great damage to a marriage. It is an addiction which requires a steady increase in severity to satisfy its viewers. Our best protection from its offensive attack on us is to defend ourselves and our homes. We are bombarded with much that we have no control over, but we do have protective power over our homes and what we see and experience there.

WALKING ON THE EDGE

There are many famous last words by which people are known. As people get themselves involved in entanglements outside of marriage, they find themselves trying to cover their steps with words, actions, and deceit. In dealing with these people it has been my experience that they seldom admit to wrongdoing even when confronted with damaging evidence. Although in the early days of my ministry I was prone to accept their excuses, experience has taught me the wisdom of the adage, "If it looks like a duck, walks like a duck, and quacks like a duck, it is almost certainly a duck."

I remember confronting a male leader in our church three times regarding his relationship with a female friend of the family. Indignant, he denied any wrongdoing and uttered his famous last words, "We're just friends." With the help of an elder in the church, and at the request of his suspicious wife, I decided to get to the heart of the matter. You can imagine his reaction when we discovered him and his "friend" in a fond embrace. I'll never forget the expression on his face when he looked up and saw us standing over them. All I could say as we turned to walk away was, "Okay, now deny it!"

Some people insist on always walking right on the edge of disaster. They may protest with those famous last words, "Don't worry, nothing will happen." When I was a boy back in Southwestern Michigan, we used to spend our summer afternoons playing along the banks of Buck Creek. It was a muddy old creek, but we loved to go there and catch frogs and anything else that crawled or croaked. Like boys everywhere, as we walked along the muddy creek bank, we always wanted to get as close to the water as possible. I learned early that if you walk along the side of a muddy creek bank long enough, you will eventually fall all the way in.

The same holds true with people and their relationships with close family friends. If we place ourselves in situations which could cause the strongest man to wobble, we had better plan on getting a little muddy and very wet.

Someday, somewhere, our feet are going to slip, and we all know what it's like to try to get back on balance once we've started to fall. We grab for anything and everything in sight and wind up pulling it all in with us. Because the deceit in this type of relationship usually affects many family members, everyone winds up dirtied by it.

Regardless of the dangers in such relationships, there are those who continue to pursue them. Their famous last words might be, "We're so much in love, it must be God's will." I seriously doubt whether either party is in a position to understand what true love is. With their attraction to each other and the excitement of their new relationship they can only view it from the wrong perspective. If they could view themselves through the eyes of God and those around them, they would be less likely to feel so sure about their actions.

I think the taste of "forbidden fruit" often poisons people much like the apple into which Snow White bit. These people fall into a sleep of the will, unable to be aroused without the righteous awakening of their souls.

I was raised in a family with three brothers and two sisters. Although we were not rich, we always had enough food for everybody in the family. But even with fresh apples always in the house, there was a variety I much preferred that grew in an orchard not far from our neighborhood. Having been neglected for years, the apples were not that tasty. Instead, their flavor came from the exciting experience of pilfering them. And so it is with the forbidden fruit outside of marriage: It is the excitement more than the fruit itself that draws the thief back for more.

Poisoned by their actions, couples even try to give the credit for their relationship to God. Perhaps their partners were not the spiritual giants they thought they should be, so God surely would want them to establish a godly home for themselves. Those using this excuse need to be aware that God has made it clear in His Word that any extramarital involvement is sin, and that's that!

USEFUL AGAIN

Although I have shared principles which can help keep unnecessary stress out of your marriage, I am aware that many readers find themselves the victims of bad choices they have already made in their past. If you have experienced the trauma of divorce, premarital sex, or extramarital sex, you need to 1) confess your share of the blame to God, and 2) turn from any repetition of the sin.

Having achieved the above, put all guilt behind you and get busy serving God. God will forgive you and use you just as you are. Remember, He reached down and brought healing to King David in spite of all that he had done, and He continued to use him throughout the rest of his life.

But there is a special caution to those who are presently involved in some kind of relationship outside of marriage: *Turn from your sin before you try the patience of God and are brought to public shame,* as King David was. God stands waiting with arms wide open to receive all His children who seek forgiveness, anxious to restore them.

It is God's will that we daily use the gifts He has given us. If your gifts are shelved because of previous sin in your life that has been forgiven, take those gifts off the shelf right now and open them up for God's use once again!

6

STRESSED-OUT KIDS

Children are an unusual gift from heaven. They can bring their parents unmatched joy and yet at the same time cause frustration, pain, and stress unlike anything the parents have ever known before. This is clearly seen when a child is missing. When the reality that the child cannot be found hits home, a fear that is difficult to describe grips the parents' hearts.

The other day I ran into our neighbors as they frantically searched for their six-year-old daughter who had not returned home from school that day. For two hours they had been retracing her route home from school. By now fear was written all over their faces. Fortunately this story had a happy ending: Their daughter was found playing happily in *our* backyard, totally unaware of the incredible stress she was putting on her parents. When she got home from school that day, my children had invited her to play, and she simply forgot to check in at home first.

Overwhelmed with relief upon finding her lost child, the mother scooped her daughter up into her arms, weeping with joy just to know that no harm had come to her. Later she followed up with some helpful reprimands to help her daughter realize why her parents were so distressed.

BULLETPROOFING OUR KIDS?

A recent magazine article entitled "Is the World Safe for Children Today?" reflects the unstable atmosphere in which today's children are growing up. Coupled with the fear of gang violence, shattered homes, and the prevalence of illegal drugs, our children face a hostile world which can cause them to crack under the stress.

It was recently reported on the evening news that the newest back-to-school accessory in New York City is the "bulletproof school jacket" to protect children from errant bullets as they walk to and from school. My memories of trips back and forth from school are of kicking the leaves that had fallen or of racing home to see who could run the fastest. But times have changed, and our children are being forced to face a much more stressful world than ever before.

Stress begins early for America's children. Many as young as two years old are dropped off at six a.m. to put in a 12-hour day at the local daycare center. Parents often tend to have high expectations of their children's abilities to read early. Many times these children are made to feel like failures if they are unable to perform above average by the time they begin their elementary education. Perhaps our expectations would be different if we could picture kindergarten as a garden where little seeds are planted and watched over, then watered with love and extra care to prepare them to survive the rigors to come. If these little budding plants are not protected from the stress of overexpectations and categorization, they may not be able to develop as they should, and some may not survive at all.

Children will face these stresses soon enough as they pass through their later years of schooling. They will feel it from their parents, teachers, and friends. How can we as parents tell whether our children are under more pressure than they can handle? What can we do to help relieve some of the stresses our children are suffering?

OUT OF THE COCOON

Although change follows children of all ages, it jumps into high gear as children hit their teen years. Parents can see changes occur almost daily as the dawn of puberty strikes. Children with "peaches-and-cream" complexions change appearance as their faces become covered with acne. One morning he or she comes out to breakfast and we no longer see a child sitting across the table from us. He doesn't look, sound, or act the same. Not only do our kids' clothes no longer fit, but they no longer see how their parents fit into their lives.

As if this weren't enough, while trapped in this precarious state they are called upon to make decisions which will affect them for the rest of their lives. While they are grappling with the realities of puberty, everyone wants to know what they intend to be when they grow up. If the truth were known, most kids have spent more time thinking about what they will wear to school tomorrow than what they plan to do with the rest of their lives.

Now enter the dating years. What a gut-wrenching experience that is! Even the most self-confident young man worries about the outcome of asking a girl for a date. Meanwhile, worried girls sit nervously waiting for the phone call that may never come.

Finally boy meets girl, girl gets boy, and the real fun begins. Mom and Dad enjoy getting to know their child's steady, and then someone new enters the picture. The song is true, "Breaking Up Is Hard to Do." Both families experience the pain of the severed relationship as their offspring feel like their worlds have come to an end. And then a new boyfriend or girlfriend enters the picture and the fun starts all over again!

Each step we take as we walk through life with our children takes them a little closer to their final destination of independence. The teenage years are much like the transitions which a caterpillar encounters as it matures into a beautiful and independent butterfly. Not all the stages are pleasant, but they are all necessary for maturation.

It is quite natural for teenagers to struggle to free themselves from the tight-fitting cocoon which seems to entomb them. What before was a safe haven protecting them from the world outside now seems to weigh them down and entrap them. Although we may want to try to help our teenagers get through this struggle painlessly, we cannot. The struggle is part of the process that strengthens their independence and prepares them for solo flight. As the butterfly wrestles to free itself from the cocoon, it is gaining the strength in its wings which will make flying possible. As your child wrestles free from your protection, he too is gaining the strength necessary for solo flight.

We as parents can do much to protect our children from unnecessary stresses which complicate the process. With the Bible as our guide we can enter and exit this period of time in the lives of our children with confidence and contentment.

CHAIN OF COMMAND

Ephesians 6:1-3 states God's chain of command for the family: "Children, obey your parents in the Lord, for this is right. Honor your father and mother, which is the first commandment with promise: that it may be well with you and you may live long on the earth." Two separate commands are given, followed by two consequences for those who obey them.

The first of the two commands deals with the proper action to take: Children are to obey their parents. This is part of God's chain of command for all His creation. We are told that citizens are to obey those who have authority over them, namely, their governments. Employees are to be in submission to and obey their employers. Wives are to be in submission to and obey their husbands, and husbands are to cherish their wives. God established chains of command throughout His creation to minimize chaos and anarchy in society, government, and the home.

Rare is the occasion when parents ask children to commit acts which violate God's Word, but that contingency is covered by the phrase that children are to obey their parents in the Lord.

The short phrase "in the Lord" is a safety net designed by God to protect children from wrongdoing. This is consistent with the command to obey those in government who have authority over us. When the apostle Peter was forced to choose between disobeying God or disobeying those governing the land, he was quick to obey God even though it meant disobeying the government. Peter obeyed the government "in the Lord," but ceased when the government failed to govern "in the Lord."

The text also explains *why* children should obey their parents. In addition to being the *right* thing to do, it is also the *smart* thing to do! God says that it will lead to a longer and more pleasant life and a home that is free of some of the most unpleasant stresses that families endure.

IS YOUR HOME A STRESS CENTER?

Unfortunately, a child's most dominant stresses usually occur within what ought to be the security of his home and family. In 1984, Charles Lewis, M.D., under the auspices of the UCLA Research Facility, did a study of stress in fifth- and sixth-graders. The children being studied were asked to compile a list of the circumstances that made them feel the most worried, depressed, or stressed. Interestingly, three of the four most common responses involved their relationship with their parents, with their greatest fear being the separation of their mom and dad. This was followed by pressure from peers to do or try something they didn't want to do. Number three was having their parents argue in front of them. Number four was the lack of time with Mom and Dad.

Thomas Boice, M.D., Director of the Child's Study Unit of the University of California, San Francisco Medical Center, observed regarding the findings, "The item that stood out to me on this list was 'not spending enough time with Mom and Dad.' On the adult list of kid-stressors it probably would have been left out, but for kids this is so important."

Parents need to be sensitive to unusual behavior in their children and be prepared to help them cope with the unique stresses they face.

CLUES TO TOO MUCH STRESS

Experts tell us that certain physical and emotional symptoms can provide clues to when a person is struggling with too much stress. The following are the ten most recognizable:

1. Tense muscles; sore neck, shoulders, and back; tension in the body.
2. Insomnia; inability to sleep or to stay asleep.
3. Unexplained fatigue.
4. Boredom, depression, listlessness, dullness, or lack of interest in things.
5. Drinking too much.
6. Eating too much or too little.
7. Unexplained diarrhea, cramps, gas, or constipation.
8. Abnormal heartbeat or palpitations of the heart.
9. Unexplained phobias.
10. Tics, restlessness, or itching.

The symptoms listed above can indicate the presence of dangerous stress in all people, regardless of age.

The study then continued by listing physical and behavioral clues that a child may be under abnormal pressure and stress. Although every child will exhibit some of the following symptoms at one time or another, parents should become concerned when the clues hit in bunches or are continual.

Physical signs:

1. Headaches
2. Stomachache
3. Trembling

4. Nervous tics
5. Teeth-grinding or complaints of a sore jaw
6. A rise in accident-proneness
7. Frequent urination or bed-wetting

Behavioral signs:

1. Crankiness and laziness
2. Anxiety
3. Nervousness
4. Poor eating habits
5. Excessive TV-watching
6. Sleeping problems
7. Nightmares

If your child is experiencing several of the above or if one of them is frequent or severe, you would be wise to investigate his or her daily schedule to see what might be causing the problem. Many times the problems are health-related, so don't hesitate to contact your family doctor.

Stress intensifies as changes and uncertainties occur, and, as we saw earlier, nobody faces more uncertainty and unrelenting change than a growing child.

God addressed four major realms of change in a child's life when He condensed a wealth of wisdom regarding the field of child psychology into one verse. Luke 2:52 states, "Jesus increased in wisdom and stature, and in favor with God and men." Written about Jesus when He was a 12-year-old, it reveals how He had victory in undergoing the tremendous changes He was experiencing.

MENTAL GROWTH

As a 12-year-old, Jesus was going through one of the most intense periods of intellectual discovery and learning. Even though He was the Son of God, Luke 2:52 says that Jesus "increased in wisdom."

Although intellectual growth can be exciting and stimulating it can also be extremely stressful. Children are under tremendous pressure to do well in school in order to get a good scholarship or gain admission into a top college or university. Although learning can be exciting, it can also be frustrating. This is especially true if children are not doing well with their grades in school. Parents need to be stationed close by in order to jump in and help their children deal with what they are experiencing.

One recent study which addressed student stress offered the following suggestions for parents to help their children cope with stress at school:

1. Show interest in what your children do at school. Ask them about the activities of the day.
2. Praise them for their efforts.
3. Be in touch with their teachers. Let teachers know if situations at home are adding stress to your child.
4. Don't put too much emphasis on grades.

PHYSICAL GROWTH

We read that Jesus grew not only in wisdom but also in stature. While on this earth for 33 years, Jesus was tempted in all the ways we are. He literally faced the same temptations as your 12-year-old son faces. The difference is that because Jesus is God, He never yielded to temptation.

It is important that parents take the initiative to instruct their children regarding the proper care and maintenance of their changing bodies. Just as mechanical engines will not run efficiently on junk fuel, physical bodies will not run efficiently on junk food. Parents who send their children to school with an inadequate breakfast are sending them into a competitive world with a serious handicap.

Studies show that Americans are not getting enough sleep. Growing bodies need plenty of rest to sustain continued growth. This is especially true in light of the amount of physical and intellectual exertion that children experience daily. Parents are doing their children no favors when they allow them to miss much-needed sleep. Everybody pays the price as parents attempt to drag an exhausted child out of bed and off to school the morning after a late night—all because of a television program that was probably at best a waste of time and more likely a negative influence on your child. Growing bodies and minds need lots of sleep. Don't let your children shortchange themselves.

With their physical growth comes the increased role of competition in their young lives. Competition can be good and instructive as it prepares children for an adult world which is highly competitive, but they can suffer if it is too intense or too early.

When I was in junior high school, I had a friend whose father was a frustrated baseball player. His dad had been good enough to make it to the minor leagues, but like thousands of other good baseball players, he didn't have that special talent to make it up to the majors. After several years of frustration he quit professional baseball and entered another profession. Not long afterward he was married and set out to raise his son. He was possessed with the aspiration of turning his son into a baseball star who could fulfill his own unrealized dreams. While the rest of the boys from the neighborhood spent the summer running through the woods or playing baseball on a rough diamond that we had carved out of an empty field, my friend was forced to pitch to his dad in the backyard. This went on day after day and week after week. Unfortunately, as he grew older, the son resisted his dad's pushing and turned against his father's dream.

SOCIAL GROWTH

In addition to His intellectual and physical growth, Jesus grew socially. Luke 2:52 says, "Jesus increased in wisdom and stature, and in favor with God and men." His social growth involved His ability to "grow in favor with men."

Do you remember how powerful peer pressure was when you were in junior high school? You dressed like your friends, you talked like your friends, and you listened to the same music as your friends. Because of the powerful pressure to conform, few teenagers are willing to truly stand out in a crowd. Their peers replace their parents as the people by whom teens most want to be accepted. The fear of being different or rejected haunts all but the most self-assured of teenagers.

These same teenagers are just beginning the "great American dating ritual." I can remember to this day the stress I faced the first time I asked a girl out for a date. It took me ten attempts before I had the courage to finish dialing her complete telephone number. I kept inventing reasons to hang up and try again later. In truth, I was haunted by the fear that she would reject my overture.

While young men grapple with the icy fear of being turned down, the girls wonder if a boy will ever call their number or whether they will end up an unwanted old maid. And of course they also face the trauma of being asked out by one of those boys with whom no respectable girl ever wants to be seen in public.

And that's just the beginning of the stress. Girls fret over whether they're too short or too tall, too skinny or too fat. Meanwhile the guys spend hours in front of the bathroom mirror trying to spot the first trace of facial hair so they can shave it off. Guys and girls alike face the stress of waking up on the morning of the biggest date of their young lives only to faint in front of the mirror when they discover a new crop of "zits" that set in during the night!

An especially harsh aspect of their social growth is the pain of being dumped by a boyfriend or girlfriend. Parents need to remember that the child is going through a pain equivalent to the pain of divorce. Both involve extreme social rejection.

As teenagers try to navigate through these difficult years, they turn to others for help. Unfortunately, they usually turn to their peers who are in the midst of the same struggles. They need their parents now more than ever, but parents must be persistent and tactful in the way they offer assistance, whether it be solicited or volunteered. Above all, parents must never desert their kids during the tumultuous teen years. Their social world is in constant flux, and they need a safe haven to turn to when they run out of answers.

Spiritual Growth

I will not even attempt to explore the theogical ramifications of God the Son growing in His relationship with God the Father. Suffice it to say that for the purpose of this study, according to God's Word in Luke 2:52, as a 12-year-old boy "Jesus grew in favor with God."

Jesus was at the age that finds many kids struggling with life-changing spiritual questions which will have a profound impact on the rest of their lives. I was raised in the church, and like so many others, I accepted Christ as my Savior at an early age. But like so many kids who have been raised in evangelical churches, I came to a point in my teens when I needed the beliefs of my parents and church to become my own. I began to feel the weight and impact of my sins through the convicting love of the Holy Spirit.

Most people set their spiritual course for life during their teen years. It is imperative that they be exposed to excellent Christian role models during their junior and senior high years. Parents cannot afford to wait for their church to develop a dynamic youth program; their kids may be gone before that it happens. Parents need to get involved with a church that has a youth program which will draw their kids toward Christ and not away from the church. Too many churches get kids saved at an early age, but due to the lack of an aggressive youth program stymie their growth toward Christian maturity.

Many young adolescents wrestle with insecurity regarding their salvation. Because they were saved at a young age, they can barely remember the details. They grow worried every time they hear the testimony of a Christian who was saved as an adult after a life of drunkenness and debauchery. The child can't remember how his life changed substantially when he was saved as a nine-year-old, and so he wonders if he is really saved. Many are the nights he lies awake in bed "accepting Christ" again in an attempt to "do it right this time." This is an excellent time for parents to talk through the salvation process with their teens and to lead their child to Christ if there is any uncertainty.

TRUE HONOR

After being told to obey, children are commanded in Ephesians 6:2 to honor their parents. Whereas to obey is the action, to honor is the attitude which should lie behind the action. This principle is ageless in its application. Whether we are 16 or 60, we are instructed to maintain an attitude of honor toward our parents. Here are some of the important aspects of true honor.

1. *Respect.* A child who honors his parents will show them respect. He will respect what they have to say and heed their warnings about potential dangers in life.

2. *Trust.* Children who honor their parents will trust them. There are few people in this world whom you can trust without reservation to have your best interests in mind. In normal situations, your parents are among those few who are truly concerned for your welfare.

    In mountain climbing, a rope is attached to the various climbers for their own safety. Each climber benefits from those climbing ahead of him. They know which path holds danger and which will bring safety. The climber just ahead of you is 25 feet beyond you in the climb and has stepped on all the rocks which you are now searching for.

    Our fathers are attached to us by a rope of love. They

climb 25 years ahead of us and experience much of the dangerous and slippery footing we are about to encounter. Even as we grow into mid-life, our fathers remain just that far ahead of us in experience and wisdom. It's healthy for our children to see *us* seeking help and advice from our *own* parents, for this builds the foundation of family trust.

3. *Values.* Character is best described as what a person is like in private when no one else can see him. One of the surest tests of whether a child honors his parents is how much he obeys his parents when they are not around.

   I can think of no finer examples of such obedience than Shadrach, Meshach, Abednego, and Daniel. These four Jewish youths were about 14 years old when they (and approximately 70 other young men) were taken as captives to the city of Babylon by King Nebuchadnezzar. They were not there long before they faced a crisis which threatened their lives. They were told that as part of their training program, they would be fed the best food available in Babylon. (Most of the citizens would have jumped at the opportunity to dine on the king's food.) The problem was that the food had been offered to idols, and God's Word told them that this was strictly off-limits. They had been taught this by their parents since they could first remember, but they could have chosen to violate their parents' values because their parents would never find out. At the risk of challenging the king, Shadrach, Meshach, Abednego, and Daniel requested food that would not only keep them healthy but would fit into the requirements of their faith.

   As the four honored their parents' values, they honored their parents. The test came when their parents were not around and would never discover what they did. Shadrach, Meshach, Abednego, and Daniel passed one of life's most difficult tests.

4. *Time.* Although I have yet to experience personally the loss of a parent, on many occasions I have performed funerals for friends who have just lost a parent. Many are the times I have heard adult children lament because they had so much wanted to share with the deceased

parent but never took the time in their busy schedule to do so—and now it was too late.

If we are fortunate enough to have our parents still alive, we need to honor them with our time. Even though they may live too far away for frequent visits, we can use the telephone more frequently. And we need to remember to bring the children to visit their grandparents for it gives them the opportunity to visit with their living legacy. Years truly do fly by, and we don't want to wake up one day to realize that we have lost forever the chance to express how much we care for the ones who helped make us who we are. One of the surest tests to determine whether we honor another person is seen by the amount of time we spend with him or her.

5.   *Support.* I believe in the responsibility of children to take care of their elderly parents, and especially their widowed mothers. First Timothy 5:8 says, "If anyone does not provide for his own, and especially for those of his household, he has denied the faith and is worse than an unbeliever." The context of the passage deals with the family's responsibility in taking care of its needy members. In situations where there is no immediate family, the church is to care for their needs. In so doing, we honor our parents and elders. Unfortunately, the majority of evangelical churches today have failed to demonstrate this form of honor.

Every now and then I read some article which calculates the frightening amount of money that experts say it will cost me to raise each of my five children. It sounds like more than I'm planning on actually making during the time they're at home! What is equally alarming is the cost of caring for elderly parents in poor health. With people living longer, the children we are investing in today may become our caretakers tomorrow. As they say, "What goes around comes around." Someday my wife and I might show up on our children's doorsteps and announce that it is now our turn to collect!

THE PROMISES

Quality and quantity of life are promises for those who obey and honor their parents. Ephesians 6:1,2 declares that this is the first commandment with promise. The promise is contained in verse 3, which states, "That it may be well with you and you may live long on the earth."

The first of the two promises involves the quality of life and is evidenced in the words "that it may be well with you."

Many homes are war zones. Battles rage as children refuse to obey their parents or submit to their authority, while others simply yield to superior strength. Everyone in the home feels the stress level rise as the child disobeys and dishonors his parents. They are left with no recourse other than discipline, which causes the tension in the home to rise still further.

It is important for children to realize that their disobedience is usually the principal cause of disharmony in the home. God makes it very clear that obedience leads to peace and harmony in the home, whereas disobedience forces godly parents to chasten the child they love. When this occurs nobody is happy, and peace escapes the family.

When they hear about children who push their parents on every rule, some parents smugly assume that it is because these parents have failed to properly discipline the child. After all, their precious darlings have done everything their parents have ever requested since the day they were born.

Let me assure you that not all children are created equal! Parents who have never experienced the challenge of raising a strong-willed child have little understanding of the magnitude of the challenge. These are special kids who have the potential to do incredible service for the cause of Christ and who likely will excel in whatever field they choose to pursue, but in the meantime they will test their parents' patience despite the best of plans.

Ephesians 6:3 lists a second consequence for children who obey and honor their parents: "That you may live long on the earth." Does this really mean what it sounds like—that children who honor and obey their parents will live longer than those who fail to honor and obey? *Quantity* of life is exactly what it means!

We often gloss over portions of Scripture telling what a heinous sin it is for children to be disrespectful toward any of their elders, but especially toward their parents. But God's Word makes His reaction to such behavior graphically clear. This is typified in the story about the prophet Elisha in 2 Kings 2:23,24: "He went up from there to Bethel; and as he was going up the road, some youths came from the city and mocked him, and said to him 'Go up, you baldhead! Go up, you baldhead!' So he turned around and looked at them, and pronounced a curse on them in the name of the Lord. And two female bears came out of the woods and mauled forty-two of the youths." Kids, be very careful to give your elders due respect and honor!

ALL IS NOT LOST

Much has been written criticizing America's teenagers, but I am still convinced that our nation will be in capable hands when our offspring move into positions of leadership in the coming years.

My confidence is supported by a recent study conducted on the 24,000 high school seniors listed in the annual copy of *Who's Who in U.S. High Schools*. The profile that emerged of these student leaders is reassuring. Fifty-two percent of them watch less than ten hours of television per week. Seventy-six percent have never engaged in premarital sex. Eighty-eight percent have never even tried a cigarette. Ninety-four percent have never as much as sampled any form of drug, including marijuana. Seventy-one percent of our future "movers and shakers" take the time to attend church regularly.

I can assure you that in almost all the cases listed above, the parents were actively involved in the lives of their children. Parents *do* make a difference!

A. R. Adams conducted a study of stress among children and came up with the following observations. He concluded, first and foremost, that if parents want intelligent and well-adjusted kids, they must keep the home strong and the marriage together. When we study children or adults with serious behavioral problems, we almost always find a dysfunctional marriage in the child's background. Seldom do deeply disturbed children emerge from situations where they live with both biological parents in a harmonious home. When marriages break down, the children will invariably pay some of the consequences.

Many of you are presently attempting to raise one or more children without the benefit of a spouse. You have already experienced the trauma of a divorce, and unfortunately your kids are still struggling to adjust. You can't change what has already happened in your life, but you can commit to raising your kids as God would have you. I can assure you that God honors the efforts of a single parent to raise godly children.

FOLLOW THE PLAN!

The Adams survey also found that when there was significant stress in the home, I.Q. scores dropped an average of 13 percent. Family stress caused kids to lose interest in both school and personal values.

Adams concluded by noting, "High achievers and law-abiding people come from homes where both parents are present and have religious influence in the home." In other words, if parents follow the plan that God ordained for them, their home will be spared many of the stresses that plague families across our land.

The same principle applies to children: If children follow God's plan by obeying and honoring their parents, they will live long on the earth and will be spared the stress of living in a home torn apart by disharmony and dishonor.

7

When Parents Panic

Upon occasion I have the opportunity to teach graduate classes at a local university. My favorite class explores the philosophical foundations of American education, and is taken primarily by public school teachers. Among the questions I ask my students is, From their experience in the classroom, which factor is most crucial in determining how well a child will do not only in school but in life? Will it be how much money the child's family possesses, or where they live? Will it be their ethnic heritage, or the number of students in the class, or some other factor?

Having taught this particular class many times before, I know beforehand how my students will respond: They will always agree that it is the *parents* who most determine how a child will do in school specifically and in life in general. Although other factors will either enhance or diminish a child's emotional, educational, social, and spiritual development, Mom and Dad are the first and foremost "twig benders" in a child's life.

A Mother's Kiss

Trees are marvelous examples of God's creation. They provide us with shade from the heat of the sun, shelter from the cold winds that blow, and fruit and nuts to ease our hunger. Extracts from trees give us rubber, lumber, and many other useful products. Beginning life as frail twigs, trees bend easily to the wind to avoid breaking. When the winds blow constantly in one direction, a tree may develop a permanent bent in that direction. It may break with severe winds, but it will not bend the other way.

Consider the case of the famous painter Benjamin West. When he was a child his mother asked him to watch his baby sister,

85

Sally, while Mom ran some errands. While she was gone, young Benjamin discovered some bottles of ink in one of the cupboards and thought how nice it would be to paint a picture of baby Sally for mother. True to form, he not only got ink on the paper but also on Sally, the floor, and himself. Try to imagine Mom's reaction as she walked into that ink-splattered living room. After quickly assessing the situation, and without exploding, she bent down to her son and with love in her voice said, "Why, Benjamin, you've painted a picture of Sally!" She then gave him a loving kiss. Years later when he was a successful painter, West stated, "My mother's kiss made me a painter." Any other reaction might have stifled the creativity of her child. She used the opportunity to bend the twig just right, and as the twig was bent, so grew the tree.

THE TRUE PROVING GROUND

Churches today are experiencing the breakdown of the family unit at almost the same ratio as the world. We are seeing more and more children brought up in homes where survival is the name of the game, and shaping and molding comes only when Mom or Dad have the energy or desire to share it.

Even in positions of leadership within the church we are not getting the proper exemplary behavior we need. When God lists the qualifications of the men who are to lead His church, He highlights the home as the key proving ground. First Timothy 3:1-7 gives us the qualifications a man must have to be an elder (or pastor). A leader must be "one who rules his own house well, having his children in submission with all reverence, for if a man does not know how to rule his own house, how will he take care of the church of God?"

One of the failures in recent years among evangelical churches has been their acceptance of men into positions of leadership who do not qualify in this area. Whether desperate for a leader or choosing to wink at God's standard for leadership, they install unqualified men in positions of great authority, with potentially disastrous results. Inevitably, shortcomings which lead to disharmony between a man and his wife and children will lead to disharmony within any church he is allowed to lead.

As a parent I realize that children do not come with a "how-to manual" for success. It is a learn-as-you-go endeavor. Parents will make mistakes, and God does not expect perfection in our homes—only adherence to His principles of obedience, worship, and service.

DO NOT PROVOKE

Ephesians 6:4 states, "Fathers, do not provoke your children to wrath, but bring them up in the training and admonition of the Lord." Approaching the Bible as a compendium on child psychology, we can use its illustrations and elaborations as divine principles for rearing godly children. There are two aspects to the above commandment, one positive and the other negative.

The first instruction is negative, telling us what to avoid. Although our English translations say, "*Fathers*, do not provoke your children to wrath," the Greek word is used elsewhere in the New Testament to refer to *parents* (Hebrews 11:23 is one such example). *Both* parents are cautioned against provoking their offspring to anger or wrath.

Having said this, I must add that fathers are most often guilty of provoking wrath within their children and should carefully heed the biblical warning. Colossians 3:21 contains a very similar instruction: "Fathers, do not provoke your children, lest they become discouraged." We need to beware of breaking the spirit of a child by discouraging him or frustrating the spirit of creativity and zeal within him.

What exactly is it that parents do to cause wrath to ferment in the tender hearts of their children? Here are some of the chief causes of wrath in children. Some of them are done unknowingly, while others are committed by parents fully aware of what they are doing. These wrath-builders are neglect, cruelty, overexpectation, favoritism, overprotection, and threats.

NEGLECT

It is no secret that children crave and thrive on attention. In their early years they are constantly seeking approval and attention from their parents, with repercussions for Mom and Dad if it is not given. Our willful neglect of our children to promote our own needs and wants can cause great anger in the heart of a child.

Recently a friend shared with me how he had been asked by his adult sons to play golf with them. He tearfully expressed his amazement that they even wanted to spend time with him. During the years they were growing up he seldom took the time to play with them, always putting other activities before spending time with his sons. He felt very fortunate that they could forgive him and reach out not in wrath but in love.

The Bible records a number of cases of child neglect and the resulting wrath. Three thousand years ago a boy named Absalom was raised in a wealthy and powerful family. His father was David, King of the nation of Israel. David was so busy ruling an empire that he neglected to spend the time with Absalom that the boy craved and needed. This father's neglect resulted in a son filled with wrath toward both David his father and life in general. Absalom rebelled against his dad and sought to take his kingdom from him, finally getting the attention he sought from his father.

CRUELTY

God, who understands child psychology much better than human experts on the subject, knows that well-placed and properly timed physical correction will do children good and not harm. Like so many other things, discipline which is designed to be positive and of great value to the child can be taken to an extreme in the hands of undisciplined parents. There is never an intention of cruelty when the Bible says, "Spare the rod and spoil the child." Unfortunately, there are parents who use this concept as a license to inflict harsh words or cruel punishment on their children.

Verbal cruelty toward a child can provoke wrath and anger just as easily as physical abuse. I'm sure most of us have listened to an angry parent verbally lash out at his or her child and call him names he would never call another human being. I've listened as a father returns home from a brutal day at work and with the least provocation turns his frustration loose on those who can't retaliate . . . his children. The attack may be merely verbal, but the wrath provoked within the hearts of the children will be just as tangible as if they had been struck physically.

We need to take special care to avoid cruel words in front of a child's peers. When a parent invades a child's sphere of friends and proceeds to embarrass him in front of them, the guaranteed result will be a simmering wrath within the child.

Needless to say, all the above cautions also apply to the use of *physical* correction of children. Spanking ought to be as painful for the parent as it is for the child. It needs to be an expression of a loving parent caring for the well-being of an erring child. Discipline done in anger and violence, inflicting possible physical and emotional harm, is counterproductive. Instead of bringing our children to a place of willing submission, this kind of abuse forces them to build walls, confusing their feelings toward us and our authority over them.

We want them to learn to obey us with a respectful but loving fear of our authority, backed up by consistent discipline. This type of discipline and the ability to submit to it make it easier for our children to understand the healthy fear we are to have of God, and His rightful authority over us.

OVEREXPECTATION

There is nothing wrong with children acting like children. After all, that is what they are! Even though your ten-year-old may surprise you at times with a statement worthy of the most mature adult, the very next minute may find him behaving like a five-year-old. This phenomenon continues and intensifies as children enter the teen years. When it comes to correction, we need to be careful to discern between willful disobedience and mere childishness. Our children may do things which we consider to be silly, but frankly, there are things we do which I'm sure the kids feel are crazy! Let's just let the kids act their age and pick our battles carefully. We want to use discipline for character-building and not demolition.

FAVORITISM

Jacob and Esau must have been quite a challenge for their parents. Their sibling rivalry began even before birth, as they struggled within the womb. Unfortunately, their parents aggravated the problem by taking sides in their squabbles. As if grabbing two sides of a wishbone and pulling it apart, Mom favored Jacob while Dad favored Esau.

I find my attention drawn in different directions by our five very different children. Realizing that it is imperative that they all feel equally loved by their dad, I am careful to avoid statements which would breed the belief that I favor one child at the expense of the others. I have to beware of statements which force comparisons, such as, "Why can't you get good grades like your sister?" or "Your brother never gets in trouble at school."

Children may even view frequent compliments aimed at one

of their friends as nothing more than a personal put-down. Depending on his or her personality, each child will respond differently to a parent's attentions, whether positive or negative. Properly evaluating each child's temperament can give you the freedom to handle each situation on the basis of how that particular child will respond.

OVERPROTECTION

My natural instinct as a father is to protect my children from any and all harm. They will always be my "babies" even if they grow to be twice my size. Unfortunately, this perfectly natural and well-meaning parental instinct can cause children to resent attentions if taken too far. We live in a cruel world which is inhabited by sinful people. Although we may be able to delay the time when our children face life alone, we will not be able to prevent it. One day they must learn how to hold down a job, pay their own bills, and settle their own squabbles.

It is natural for young adults to want to be in control of their own lives. I agree with the statement, "It is better to risk too much trust in a child than too much protection." I would rather have my children learn the sting of failure while they are still under my roof, where I can help them discover how to correct their errors. I don't want them facing their first life-changing decision when they are 18 years old and lacking any experience in knowing how to make proper choices.

Upon entering college most young adults begin to question things they have been taught about their faith and standards. This is a very natural part of the maturation process. What had been their parents' stand on issues must either become their own by choice and conviction, or be rejected because they as individuals cannot defend it. Parents who wisely allowed their children latitude in some important decision-making while at home actually give their children the advantage of not having to learn how to make decisions after they have left.

THREATS

Kids must be assured that parental love is not dependent upon their behavior. Statements like "Mommy won't love you if you don't come in on time" or "I told you so" sound like the responses coming from the mouth of a four-year-old and not a parent. Because we are to be their "city of refuge" in the midst of battle, we must never seal the door of our love, leaving them standing outside.

Children who have gone through the agony of the divorce of their parents often feel the loss of love even more dramatically. They may be led to believe deep down inside that they are responsible in some way for the hostilities at home and the separation of their parents. Little shoulders carry the guilt that even adults find too heavy. This is especially prevalent when the kids are bounced back and forth between parents and hear comments about how much of a hassle they are for their parents. Frustration and insecurity are often displayed as anger toward one or both parents. It is not uncommon for children to play the parents against each other, with full knowledge of the stress and grief it causes.

TRAINING TRUE MARKSMEN

Psalm 127:3-5 states, "Behold, children are a heritage from the Lord, the fruit of the womb is His reward. Like arrows in the hand of a warrior, so are the children of one's youth. Happy is the man who has his quiver full of them; they shall not be ashamed, but shall speak with their enemies in the gate."

I'm afraid the children of our day are growing up with confused images of the value of their existence. With abuse running rampant and abortion killing more than a million of our children yearly, what are they to believe as to their worth? How can we raise children strong in the knowledge of their abilities, who obey us out of love and respect, with such poor examples all around them?

The kind of worth we want to instill in our children today, which involves the positive transfer of values and experiences from parent to child, can be accomplished only by teaching, admonishing, and leading them in the ways of God. This positive view of instruction is found in the second half of Ephesians 6:4. We are to "bring them up in the training and admonition of the Lord."

The word "admonition" comes from a Greek word which means "a verbal instruction with a view toward correction." It means to verbally correct and alter the paths of our children as they move through life's experiences. We as parents, much like marksmen teaching their students, must show our children how to hold and string their bow and how to prepare their arrows.

Then we must encourage them to constantly practice aiming for the bull's-eye. Parents have the opportunity to teach their children how much the bow can bend before it snaps and how to guide their vision to make their aim correct before shooting off their arrows.

CAUTION: ACTIONS AT WORK

As the saying goes, "Your actions speak so loud that I can't hear what you're saying." In other words, kids learn much better by *observation* than by *argumentation*. This holds true in many different spheres of life. If you want your child to have a happy marriage, you must personally exemplify what a happy relationship is in your own marriage. Dysfunctional marriages often produce children who themselves enter into dysfunctional relationships.

Parents who want their children to avoid the pain of drug abuse need to practice abstinence from mind-altering substances themselves. Our sermons on the evils of drugs will fall on deaf ears if the child hears them from a father who periodically gets "smashed" with various forms of alcohol or drugs.

At our church preschool, we occasionally experience a child using unacceptable language. When the child's parents are informed of the problem, they usually vow to get to the heart of the situation. Although we appreciate their commitment, we know where nine out of ten foul-mouthed preschoolers learn their words: from their parents. Children often mimic their parents down to the way they walk and the way they talk. If foul language is used freely in the home, the child will feel free to use it at his discretion, often suffering consequences that he does not understand.

The best way to raise kids who don't cheat in the classroom or on the playground is to have them daily observe parents who are honest and have personal integrity in all they do and say. Even young children learn the value of honesty when they find something that doesn't belong to them and have to seek out its owner, relinquishing their rights to it. Finders are not always keepers.

PREVENTING FUTURE GRIEF

The Bible tells us that when a father loves his child, he chastens wrongdoing. In reality, a father who fails to chasten his child hates his child. This chastening may be either physical or verbal, but if it is done with love it can help the child mature properly. If done early and consistently, it can save our children much grief in *their* lives as well as in our *own* lives.

We demonstrate our love by clearly showing our children where they have erred. By making our children accept the responsibility for their own actions, we can raise trustworthy young people. We can also teach our children to be accepting of our discipline by our own willingness to admit our errors and shortcomings.

UNTAUGHT ABILITY

Kids don't need to be taught how to sin; they figure that out all by themselves! This is proven daily in the home of every two-year-old. Left to themselves, children exhibit the sinful nature unbridled. They defy reason, tease and taunt, lie, steal, hit, and disobey without a thought for the consequences. Romans 3:23 says, "All have sinned and fall short of the glory of God." The "all" includes even the tiniest of babies. Psalm 58:3 concludes, "The wicked . . . go astray as soon as they are born." This is why God instructs us in Proverbs 13:24, "He who spares his rod hates his son, but he who loves him disciplines him promptly." What we don't want to do is send our children off as young adults still behaving like two-year-olds. That's why God has chosen to let us keep our children around for such a relatively long period of time.

Within an hour of their birth, newborn colts struggle to get up on their wobbly legs and then begin to walk. They mature at such a pace that within the first four months they are weaned from their mothers and run like the wind as they flaunt their independence.

Instead of an hour, we as parents take pride if our children can walk within the first year. And as far as kids becoming independent, it may take 18 years or longer before we send our children off on their own, many times knowing that they are still not able to stand on their own two feet emotionally, financially, and spiritually.

It is not uncommon for 16-year-olds to insist that they are completely grown up and know all they need to know to exist in the world. Just give them a driver's license and some wheels and they're ready to face just about anything . . . until the reality of insurance and the cost of gas brings them back down to earth! Many of us can vividly remember this exciting time in our lives. It's wonderful, yet it can be frightening for parents as well as kids.

We are seeing a new group of children emerge in America today. After leaving home to get married or venture out on their own career, they are discovering that life is not what they expected. The money has run out and the relationships they have been involved in have failed, leaving them with little desire to be responsible for anyone or anything. With their marriages and careers in ruin, they return home to Mom and Dad's door, sometimes with little ones trailing behind. These "bungee cord kids" are not able to support themselves financially or emotionally and need their parents' help to get their lives in order again.

Parents of these adult children are finding themselves in a difficult position of becoming their child's provider once more. This puts a new kind of stress on the parents that they don't seem to know how to handle. Their generation considered responsibility as something almost sacred, and yet they have produced children who, after struggling to free themselves of parental authority, have bounced back home again.

PRIVATE NEGLECT, PUBLIC SHAME

In Proverbs 29:15 we read, "The rod and reproof give wisdom, but a child left to himself brings shame to his mother." Many godly mothers have invested their lives in their children and will reap the return on their investment in heaven. Generations to come will be affected by what they have implanted in the hearts and minds of their sons and daughters.

In 2 Timothy 1:5 Paul pays tribute to a special mother and grandmother: "I call to remembrance the genuine faith that is in you, which dwelt first in your grandmother Lois and your mother Eunice, and I am persuaded is in you also." Paul was commending these women for the way they had raised Timothy, allowing him to experience their faith firsthand. Timothy brought great honor to them as well as to the Lord they served.

Unfortunately, there are many moms and dads out there with broken hearts and public dishonor because their children are living ungodly lives. We have all known Christian leaders who were forced to step down from their jobs and responsibilities because of the actions of their children.

LOVE AND CORRECT

Proverbs 13:24 talks about the relationship between parents and their offspring when it says, "He who loves him disciplines him promptly." In other words, correction is actually a way to show our children that we love them. Although they may not agree with this fact at the moment a spanking is being applied, or appreciate being grounded, they will someday understand the love that motivated the discipline. This realization may not come until they have children of their own and face similar questions about correction.

Hebrews 12:5-8 gives the example of true parental love when it says: "You have forgotten the exhortation which speaks to you as to sons: 'My son, do not despise the chastening of the Lord, nor be discouraged when you are rebuked by Him; for whom the Lord loves He chastens, and scourges every son whom He receives.' If you endure chastening, God deals with you as with sons; for what son is there whom a father does not chasten? But if you are without chastening, of which all have become partakers, then you are illegitimate and not sons." Applying this principle to our families, a child who is not chastened may view himself of little worth to his parents, like an illegitimate son.

Boundaries and expectations should be established by the parents and clearly understood by their children. Children should feel secure within the parameters set. Children must know that their parents want to protect them from harm that they may not be able to handle. This unspoken trust between parent and child should be their birthright and security. When parents fail to involve themselves in disciplining a child who errs, they put all the responsibility for making right and wrong choices in the lap of the unprepared child.

If we as children of God were not chastened within His love, we too would feel the insecurity of not knowing when we have crossed the boundary into danger. His gentle restraining hand reaches out and pulls us back to a place where we feel safe.

Hebrews 12:9 states that the net result of loving correction is respect: "We have had human fathers who corrected us, and we paid them respect. Shall we not much more readily be in subjection to the Father of spirits and live?" If parents demonstrate their love by consistently guiding their children with reasonable and appropriate correction, one day they will have the respect of their children. Parents who fear they will alienate their kids by disciplining them seldom end up being respected by their kids when they are grown.

MEAN WHAT YOU SAY

A threat made is a threat which must be carried out. If a child is told that failure to be at the dinner table in five minutes will mean the loss of television privileges, the penalty must be applied if the child fails to make it to the table on time. Failure to carry through consistently on correction undermines the whole process, and kids quickly learn when parents are merely blowing hot air.

This leads to all kinds of ramifications. Parents must use wisdom by not threatening punishments which are unreasonable in their length, severity, or enforcement. To ground a teenager for six months for a minor infraction takes away the parents' leverage for disciplining them later for something more serious.

It is also imperative that parents agree on the standards they expect their children to follow. Many times Mother will refuse a child's request to do something and have the situation contained, only to have her husband pipe up that he doesn't see anything wrong with what the child wants to do. The child will quickly seize the moment and drive a wedge between the two opinions. The old saying, "United we stand, divided we fall," holds true in raising children. Even though the methods may change as parents actually enter into parenting, every couple needs to discuss their differing ideas of discipline and how they want to implement them. It's hard for any child to break through this kind of united front. Then when difficult situations arise, there won't be an opportunity for children to play one parent against the other. They will already know that what one says goes for both.

MAKE YOUR STANDARDS CLEAR

Young minds certainly work differently than do those of parents; children can generalize just about any action! This is especially true with very young children. If you tell them to clean their room without specifically showing them what that involves, they will pick up a few things, thinking the room looks fine to them, and consider it a job well done. But what you wanted them to do was make their bed, pick up their toys, hang up their clothes, etc. If you tell your children what you want them to do, and even show them how you want it done, they will have a much better understanding of your exact expectations and there will be less opportunity for disagreement later.

Sometimes Dad comes home after an especially tough day at work and all he really wants is to be left alone. As he staggers into the house he is tripped up by one of the kids. He immediately flies off the handle and without thinking barks out a discipline far too harsh for a minor offense.

Called on to suffer for all the frustrations that Dad has experienced for the past eight hours, the child tries to picture in his mind what he could have done to deserve such harsh treatment. The correction is inconsistent with the offense and has no positive purpose because it is not tied to a behavior that warrants it. Being punished for innocent actions confuses the whole process in a child's mind.

CORRECT IN PRIVATE

Trips to the grocery store with small children are extremely stressful. Mom (or Dad), with grocery list in hand, wheels her way down aisle after aisle trying to find everything she needs while answering the innumerable, unanswerable questions flowing freely from her toddler's mouth. But it is when she finally gets to the checkout counter that the big battle begins. The gum, candy, magazines, and books are appropriately displayed within the child's reach. The begging begins, the tears start to flow, and the blood pressure starts to rise.

Kids seem to sense that once they are in public there is a good chance that Mom and Dad will not spank them. In a sense they are right about the wisdom of correction being handled in private.

A friend of our family felt the same way about private correction but had reached her limit with the grocery store tantrum. Finally one day she said *no* emphatically as her child continued to beg and plead in the checkout line. When there was no letup in his wailing, she excused herself and her son, explaining to the clerk her intention to return in a few minutes. With her son still crying, she walked back to her car, got inside, and explained that since he had chosen to behave in this way, even though she had said a spanking would result if he did, she had to assume he had made the choice for the spanking. She followed up on her end of the deal and returned to the store.

Still in a bit of shock, her son stopped crying, they paid for their groceries, and then they went home. After repeating the same willingness to follow through on her discipline a few more times, the crying and complaining stopped. Now going to the grocery store is something they can both enjoy, because they both know the ground rules.

Punishing a child while in the presence of his friends or other people is very threatening to both the parent and the child. Many times it blows the situation way out of proportion. It also brings embarrassment to both parties. This is why the place for discipline should be somewhat private, with only the parties involved present.

As children get older, causing them to lose face in front of their peers may not only destroy their fragile self-image but also create bitterness. Understanding the value of private correction, Jesus explained in Matthew 18:15, "If your brother sins against you go and tell him his fault between you and him alone." This principle applies not only to adults involved in church discipline but also to our children. An added benefit to seeking privacy when correcting a child is that it gives the parent a chance to cool down and gain control of his or her emotions before administering discipline.

LET THEM LEARN TO PAY

Because parents love their children and want to help them, they are often too quick to sweep up after them when they get into trouble. If your young child breaks a neighbor's window with a baseball, you may be quick to pay knowing full well that the child has no resources of his own. But as children grow older, many parents continue to step in and attempt to clean up every mess they make. Although their intentions may be good, these parents are doing their children no favors. Children need to learn early that in the real world they will be expected to make restitution when they break something.

One area where I have seen great harm done in the process of developing integrity in children is at school. When kids are confronted with unacceptable behavior, many teachers and school administrators find themselves fighting both child and parents. Many parents refuse to believe that their child is capable of doing anything wrong, and instead turn their attack on the well-meaning teacher.

It is never easy for a parent to sit on the sidelines and watch his or her child face this type of confrontation. It leads to tears, embarrassment, and sometimes expulsion. If a child has been proven to be at fault by school administrators and it reaches the point of involving the parents, the best recourse for all involved is to let the child suffer the consequences of his wrongdoing. Parents should stand together with the school and hope the lesson is well learned so that it doesn't have to be repeated.

When parents persist in stepping in to fight their children's battles, carrying the burdens of the consequences on their own shoulders instead of letting their children carry them, the whole process will repeat itself over and over again. This type of intervention teaches children to place the blame elsewhere instead of accepting responsibility for their own actions.

This principle of paying for misdeeds also applies to accepting the consequences of failure to study for exams. If your child pretends he is sick and unable to go to school (when in fact he has failed to study for an exam), it is far better to let him flunk the test and learn to plan better next time than to put your approval on this type of deceitful behavior.

KEEP YOUR PROMISES

Children must know that when promises are made they will be kept. Too many kids have learned that their parents are quick to make promises that they will keep only if it is convenient. If parents want to be able to trust the word of their children, they need to make sure that their own word can be trusted.

It is far better to refrain from making a promise than to make one that you may not be able to keep. It has always been my practice that once I have promised to do something, short of an unforeseen disaster I will do whatever it takes to deliver on my promise.

Dads, if you have told your son you will get home early from work so the two of you can play baseball, you had better make it home on time or else your word may no longer mean anything to your son. Not keeping your word to arrive at a place when you say you will is another variation of violating your word. If you truly make every effort to keep your promises, then when unforeseen circumstances prevent you from following through, those who know you will give you the benefit of the doubt.

LISTEN AND ANSWER

Kids have so many questions—everything from where peanut butter comes from to how birds fly. Sometimes even the most loving parent reaches the end of her patience and pretends to no longer hear her child's questions. On other occasions, a father may not want to be bothered by what he considers to be silly questions while he is involved in a very important project such as watching Monday Night Football . . . or Thursday night football . . . or Sunday afternoon football.

There is no such thing as a silly question when it is asked by a child. With the entire world unfolding before them, children simply have to know what is happening and why. It has been said that if parents listen to the little things now, their children will want to share the big things with them when they are older. When parents won't listen, children turn to their friends and in many cases engage in a pooling of ignorance.

PRAY . . . AND PRAY

When parents decide to bring a child into this world, they are making a decision which will affect them for the rest of their lives. One commitment they should make is to daily ask God to watch over their children. Among other things, parents should ask God to allow their children to experience what is necessary to help them grow up wanting to love and serve Him.

When our first daughter was born, a godly women reminded us that she was not ours to possess but only to care for until God wanted her back. By entrusting our children back into God's hands we can know the peace of not having to worry about them every moment of every day. Their safety is not in our hands, but in God's.

I have a cousin who served as a short-term missionary in the Philippines until conditions in that country resulted in the removal of the Campus Crusade group with which she was serving. I spoke with her mother, who had just received a letter saying that her daughter was safe and not to worry. I asked this mother how she could handle the kind of stress that accompanies not knowing whether a child is safe from danger. She replied that the only way she could handle letting her daughter go completely, without worrying every moment of the day for her safety, was to give her back to God and trust that He could take better care of her than she herself could.

I remember also talking to the daughter about how her parents were handling her comings and goings to so many countries where her safety might be in question. She shared with me that her parents told her that they had released her into God's hands, thus giving her the freedom to serve without being concerned that her parents were sick with worry.

DON'T MISS YOUR CHANCE

Proverbs 22:6 continues to stand as God's promise to parents who follow God's instructions in raising their children: "Train up a child in the way he should go, and when he is old he will not depart from it."

We all make mistakes because none of us is perfect. You may have blown it completely in raising your children, but it is never too late to change, especially if God has shown you what it is that you need to work on. Even if your children are grown, He may give you another opportunity to love and nurture your grandchildren.

Time races by so rapidly. It seems it was only yesterday that the children were born, and now look at them! One of the things I am hoping and working toward is having no regrets when my kids are raised and out of the home. I will have only one chance to be a good father, and it is my goal to be the best one I can be right now.

8

■ ■ ■ ■ ■ ■ ■ ■ ■ ■ ■ ■ ■

ON-THE-JOB STRESS

In a survey conducted by the Gallup Organization, 51 percent of the people polled said that if they could go back and start their careers over again, they would quit what they are now doing and choose different jobs. This is not too surprising when you consider how little effort people usually invest in choosing a career. According to Jim Bowe, president of Career Management Systems Inc., a Minneapolis consulting firm, "The cliche . . . and it's probably true . . . is that people spend more time planning their next vacation than they do planning what they're going to work at for the rest of their lives."

The problem is most acute when kids are in high school and should be exploring their vocational options. Most states don't require a high school student to take a career education course, and many school districts don't even have school guidance counselors. The problem is complicated by the fact that most teenagers have other things on their minds. According to Betty Olson, who owns a counseling firm in Golden Valley, Minnesota, "When you're 14, 15, 16 years old, making the team or having a date Friday night is a . . . lot more important than what you're going to do for the rest of your life."

SPECIAL FORMS OF STRESS

Our nation is filled with men and women who have been going to the same shop or office for years even though they hate their jobs. If they had it to do over again, they would choose a different career, but since they don't have it to do over again, they feel trapped. Added to this group are all those workers who are under stress because of excess pressures at work.

There are many causes of on-the-job stress. These may include

103

a boss who is always riding you. No matter what you do, it is never enough, and he is on you "like scum on a pond." Other workers face the stress of a possible layoff. During every recession in America, many workers have this stress dangling over them. Your personal stress may be from the big sale you didn't make and the big commission you won't be receiving. Or you may have just received word of an impending transfer. This wouldn't be so bad except that you bought a house last year and have no idea how to sell it without losing a bundle.

Working mothers face a special form of stress. In addition to all the normal pressures of working, many of them face guilt feelings as they drop their children off at a daycare center each morning. Others are haunted by the fear that their "latchkey" children will resent not having a mother to come home to after school. Though fully aware of such dangers, many mothers are also fully aware that they have no other choice. If they don't work, there won't be a decent house for them to live in.

Your job stress may be caused by the fact that you don't even *have* a job. Recently I received a letter from a good friend of mine in another state. After working successfully in the same industry for 17 years he was called into the boss's office and informed that he was being let go because business was sluggish. With a wife, kids, and mortgage to think about, he faces acute stress as he tries to decide what to do with his life.

Stress is a constant which can be found in every line of work. Some vocations are more severe than others, but none are spared. In my own experience of teaching at the university level, I often encounter men and women who have worked in high-powered business settings for years and have finally decided they have had enough of the pressure and the rat race. Now they are pursuing what they believe will be a stress-free career in teaching. After all, how tough could it be to spend eight hours a day with a roomful of third-graders? They'll soon find out! Each line of employment has its own unique manifestations of stress.

The wise worker, aware that on-the-job stress is unavoidable and often beyond his or her control, will seek to outsmart stress by avoiding self-induced additions to his vocational stress. I believe that the majority of job-related stresses are caused by the person suffering them. I also believe that most of the people who get fired from jobs have brought the situation upon themselves.

They have failed to follow the instructions given in the Bible on how to be both a good Christian and a good employee.

THE BIBLICAL SOLUTION

Ephesians 6:5-9 discusses the relationship between employers and their employees. To help you better understand the meaning, remember that the word "servants" can be translated "employees" and that "masters" can be translated "employers." In this passage we are given the basic principles which promote a harmonious worker/employer relationship.

"Servants, be obedient to those who are your masters according to the flesh, with fear and trembling, in sincerity of heart, as to Christ; not with eyeservice, as men-pleasers, but as servants of Christ, doing the will of God from the heart, with good will doing service, as to the Lord, and not to men, knowing that whatever good anyone does, he will receive the same from the Lord, whether he is a slave or free. And you, masters, do the same things to them, giving up threatening, knowing that your own Master also is in heaven, and there is no partiality with Him."

In these verses we see the vital principles that can help us perform our jobs with a high degree of efficiency and a much lower degree of stress. Now let's talk about these principles.

Ephesians 6:5 says that employees are to obey their employers with "fear and trembling." This is part of God's chain of command for our world. As we saw earlier, citizens are to obey those in authority over them. Wives are to obey their own husbands. Children are to honor and obey their parents in the Lord. All of these relationships are part of God's chain of command to keep this world operating without anarchy. We now read that His chain of command extends to employees and employers as well.

ARE YOU A PRODUCER?

Workers should view their jobs as a test of spiritual obedience. They are to work not only with eyeservice to please those who are watching them, but with their hearts in order to please God. We are told to do our work "as to the Lord" and "with good will." Workers who heed this command will find that they are rewarded not only by God but also by their employers. Good producers do not go unheeded for long.

Unfortunately, such producers are the exception rather than

the rule. This was made vividly clear to me while I was working my way through college. Some of the most life-changing experiences I received occurred outside the classroom as I worked at different part-time jobs. One of them was in a warehouse where, along with eight other guys, I was hired to repair damaged boxes and shipping cartons. Even though I was the new kid on the block, during the very first night I discovered that I had no trouble repacking 40 cases per hour, well over the minimum of eight that was expected by management.

As my first shift approached its end, I was taken aside by the more experienced repackers and told that I couldn't repack more than eight cases per hour. Enthusiastically I beamed that I not only could handle 40 per hour, but with a little experience I could move 50 pieces. My co-workers then sternly informed me that if I did more than eight, all the work could easily be done by half as many workers, and they would make sure I was the first to go. I later discovered that they were actually sneaking out into the warehouse and knocking over whole stacks of merchandise to assure themselves of work to do.

Some time after I left that job I learned that the management finally figured out their scam and fired the entire crew. Although it may look like people are getting away with something, eventually they will get what they deserve ... and my friends did.

That same summer I experienced the antithesis of my previous job. My new job involved selling books door-to-door. It was while I was away from home and the security of my family that I learned some of the most valuable lessons of my life. Because I didn't eat if I didn't make a sale, I worked from sunup to sundown, six days a week, for four summers. I learned the value of proper time management as I ran between houses and avoided small talk.

It was also during the summers of my college years that I learned that those who work hard and smart will be rewarded for their efforts. Working 72 hours a week was really no sacrifice when we discovered that in so doing we could make in excess of a thousand dollars a week. Not bad for college students!

THREE VITAL SECRETS

The main reason most workers get in trouble on the job is because of poor work habits. They could greatly reduce the amount of stress they face on the job if they would employ some of the basic principles of character as given in God's Word. Here are the most vital three.

1. *Dependability.* Employers love people they can depend on. When you say you will be in by 8 a.m., then be there by 8 am. and not a moment later. Don't sneak out 15 minutes early and take too much time for your lunch hour without first asking permission. Dependable workers are few and far between, and many are the companies that will gladly hire such workers.

2. *Honesty.* Be an employee who is known for honesty in all situations and with all people. American businesses fight an ongoing war against theft. Tools are stolen from shops, supplies are pilfered from offices, and merchandise is taken from stores. Contrary to what might be expected, it is not dishonest *customers* who shoplift the greatest amount of merchandise from retailers, but rather dishonest employees. There is a severe honesty crisis in America.

   Some people would never dream of stealing tangible items, but they do as much damage to their reputation by stealing something just as valuable, namely time. They call in sick even when they are well but merely want some time off. Then they justify it with the comment that "everybody does it."

   Precious is the worker whose word is gold, who can be counted on to tell nothing more and nothing less than the truth; who can be trusted around valuable merchandise without fear of theft; who can be trusted to be at work and on time unless serious illness strikes. His or her honesty will not go unnoticed by his supervisor.

3. *Irreplaceability.* A wise worker will go out of his way to learn the difficult jobs as well as those tasks that no one else wants to do. Study your industry and all that goes on in your place of employment so that you become irreplaceable. Become the person that others turn to when they don't know how something is done. Observe the work that those around you do so you can step in for them if necessary. Learn what it is that your boss does. Somebody will need to step into that position when your

boss eventually departs. Study the job above you in the corporate ladder and be ready to move up. Become the irreplaceable worker in your company. When a slow economy mandates cuts in staff, you will be the last rather than the first to receive a pink slip.

GET THAT DEGREE!

I have a close friend who always gives a day's work for a day's wage. He is one of the most dependable men I know. When he says he will accomplish a task, he does so, and on time. His honesty is beyond question. He has all of the tools to move into management at his company, but he has never been given the opportunity to show what he can do. The problem lies in the fact that he never finished college, and according to his company's policies, a college degree is a prerequisite for a position in management.

After laboring through 13 years of schooling, many young people feel the urge to take a breather from formal education before starting college. For others, their career plans do not mandate additional formal education, and that's fine. However, I have watched as those needing a college education decided to get married first, and soon they were surprised by one or more babies. Figuring they had plenty of time to get back to college, they watched the years begin to accumulate, and before long thoughts of finishing college no longer seemed feasible. Meanwhile they became locked into a dead-end job where their advancement would always be limited by their lack of a college degree.

It is never easier to attend college than immediately after high school. The foundational studies from high school are still fresh in your mind. Your obligations to other people are as limited as they will ever be. You probably don't have a spouse and children with whom you should split your time and priorities. Nor do you have a large mortgage and other debts hanging over your head like the sword of Damocles.

The friend I mentioned, who failed to complete his education, is now working faithfully to get it done. I admire his persistence and desire, and yet he and others like him would counsel their own kids to get their education as soon as possible. Waiting only leads to years of being underemployed, and efforts to complete college later on are costly in terms of time, money, and stress on the family.

DEVELOP YOUR POTENTIAL

We previously mentioned the story of Daniel, Shadrach, Meshach, and Abednego and the way they rose to positions of prominence in the Babylonian Empire—this in spite of the fact that they were Jews living in a hostile land. Modern Iraq occupies what was once the Empire of Babylon. Can you imagine four Jews being allowed to rule in modern Iraq? But these were exceptional young men of God's choosing who were filled with potential.

There are few things in life as frustrating as unused or undeveloped potential. What a waste when potential goes to waste because it has not been sharpened by a formal education! But these four Hebrew teenagers took the potential they possessed and activated it through learning. We read about part of their three years of formal training in Daniel 1:4: " ... young men in whom there was no blemish, but good-looking, gifted in all wisdom, possessing knowledge and quick to understand, who had ability to serve in the king's palace, and whom they might teach the language and literature of the Chaldeans."

From other sources we know that their training was intense and covered a broad range of learning, including the sciences, literature, languages, and more. The four young men studied diligently, and graduation day eventually arrived. We read how they did on their final exams in Daniel 1:17-20: "As for these four young men, God gave them knowledge and skill in all literature and wisdom; and Daniel had understanding in all visions and dreams. Now at the end of the days, when the king had said that they should be brought in, the chief of the eunuchs brought them in before Nebuchadnezzar. Then the king interviewed them, and among them all none was found like Daniel, Hananiah, Mishael, and Azariah; therefore they served before the king. And in all matters of wisdom and understanding about which the king examined them, he found them ten times better than all the magicians and astrologers who were in his realm."

They had activated their potential!

KEEP YOUR PRIORITIES STRAIGHT

Shadrach, Meshach, and Abednego (as well as Daniel) continued to rise through the ranks. They were so successful that their colleagues grew jealous of them and looked for a way to destroy their careers if not their lives. Their chance finally came and is recorded in Daniel 3, where we read that the king issued a decree commanding all his subjects to bow to an image of gold when they heard the sound of the musical instruments playing. Those who refused would not only be removed from office, but would be cast into a fiery furnace as well.

Needless to say, Shadrach, Meshach, and Abednego could not bow to a false god. They had their priorities straight: God came before their job. Serving God was far more important to them than their jobs or even their lives, which in His goodness God preserved for them anyway.

Stress develops when you get your priorities mixed up. When work wedges its way ahead of your marriage, children, or service to the Lord, harmony will be lost and stress will build. If your job is preventing you from being able to serve in your local church, something is wrong. Your job is stunting your spiritual maturation process and should be examined. You should not commit to a job, no matter how attractive, which prevents your involvement in a local church ministry for a prolonged period of time. Get your priorities straight.

Does your family suffer because of your job? A job which prevents you from spending quality time with your family should be reexamined to see if it has caused your family to be shoved down the priority list. Kids grow up at an incredible pace. At first it seems as if they will be around the house forever, and then one day it strikes you that they are grown now and are about to leave your home and establish their own. At this point it's too late to make up for the years of neglect caused by an all-consuming job. Don't let a job drive you out of their lives.

The same is true of your marriage. We men have been led to believe that the test of a successful husband and father is measured by the number of possessions he is able to give to his wife and children. With the best of motives young husbands work two jobs or overtime to provide *things* for their family when in reality what the family really wants and needs is *Dad at home*. One's job becomes the all-consuming passion rather than his wife and children. It isn't long before resentment builds toward both Dad and his job. The things he provides may become objects of scorn rather than love.

Keep your priorities straight and you will save yourself much future stress. Don't let your job sneak ahead of your service for God and your time with your family.

LEAVE IT AT WORK

It has been one of those days. The rush-hour traffic on the drive home was made worse by the cold drizzle. You got the word that the big sale you had been working on fell through and the boss was steamed. You ended up working late because some of the other guys called in sick and you had to finish their work. And then you walk in the front door and the kids are having a royal rumble in the front room.

Meanwhile your wife has been out shopping all day and dinner isn't ready. Just as you think things could get no worse, you answer the front doorbell, and surprise, the in-laws have decided to drop in!

All Dad now needs is the smallest of sparks to set him off. And it is likely that the spark will be provided by either his wife or his kids. As he erupts and unloads all the frustrations that built up at work, they sulk away, fearing they have done this to Dad, when in reality it was all the office problems that pushed him to the edge. He couldn't safely lash back at anyone at work without risking his job but at home he is the boss . . . or so he thinks.

A tremendous amount of stress in the home is caused by family members who don't leave their job problems at work. Rather than escaping the daily office pressures, they insist on dragging them home to the place that ought to be their safe refuge from such grief.

NAPOLEON'S SECRET

Napoleon Bonaparte was a man who seemed to thrive on pressure-packed situations. For several decades he was under a magnitude of stress which would have crushed an ordinary man. One of the ways he devised to leave his problems at "the office" was to mentally place each challenge, problem, or crisis in a separate dresser drawer and then mentally lock them. He refused to allow himself to as much as think about the problem locked in the drawer until it was time for him to solve it. This allowed Napoleon to enjoy his moments of leisure without being plagued by the stresses which accompanied his attempts to conquer the world. He knew how to leave his problems at work.

I am the only person who can ruin my day. If I choose to have a great day, try as you might to spoil it, I will have a great day. Life is really 10 percent what happens to you and 90 percent how you respond to it. Because of the nature of my ministry, I am constantly dealing with people who have lost loved ones, couples on the verge of divorce, and people facing life-shattering problems. To maintain my own sanity, I have learned that I cannot bring the problems of other people home to my family. If I do, my family will be asked to pay for the mistakes of others, and stress will result.

YOU'RE FIRED!

One of the worst fears of many workers is being called into the boss's office to hear those dreaded words, "You're fired." Let me share some observations I have made about men and women who have gone through a firing.

Most of them were not pleased with their jobs prior to being fired but were afraid to quit or even actively look for another job and thereby risk rocking an already-shaky boat. With a normal load of bills and a family to support, they didn't want to lose the bird in the hand while they searched for the two in the bush. They never would have actively sought a better job while they were still employed, but getting fired changed all that and gave them the freedom to seek a job that better suited them. Most of the fired people I have observed end up with better-paying jobs than the ones they lost. In retrospect, they realize that their worst fear—getting fired—actually became a positive and maturing experience in their lives.

Don't bring home to your family the fear of getting fired. Remember two facts: It will only cause things to grow more stressful at home, and if the firing actually does occur, you will be free to seek a job which better fulfills your needs and aspirations.

PURSUE YOUR DREAM

Being raised in Michigan, I had many friends whose fathers worked in automobile assembly plants. Although some of them enjoyed the security of their work, others despised the monotony of the assembly line. They seemed to live for their time off and vacations. For many of them, their hate for their job was so intense that they were desperately struggling toward the day when they could retire and walk off the assembly line for the last time. How unfortunate that the best hours of their prime years were being wasted doing a job they hated!

The price they paid was high. Many of them were empty shells of men by the time they reached retirement. It was as if the fire and energy had been slowly drained from them during those wasted years of manhood. There was little zest for life left when the day came to retire.

I love my job, and if I didn't I would find one that I did. I believe it is the right of each person to do a job that he or she enjoys. People who do what they enjoy do it better than those who perform begrudgingly. There is something wrong when a person invests his or her prime years in a job which he detests.

I enjoy talking with elderly people who are soon to pass away from this life and receive their heavenly reward and have no regrets regarding their lives. As they look back across the decades, they wouldn't change a thing. Even though they didn't reach all their goals, they have no regrets because at least they went after them. I want to someday look back at my life with no regrets, confident that I had the courage to pursue my dreams.

NO REGRETS

A close friend of mine always wanted to own a restaurant. I suppose the desire first began when as a young boy he watched his father run his own small bar. After college he took a position as an administrator in a large organization and did a fine job. However, that desire to open a restaurant of his own was never far below the surface of his thinking. It kept popping up in our casual conversations. As the years passed his family continued to grow, as did his financial responsibilities. To his credit, he was an excellent administrator and continued to grow in his job. But his dream was still to open his own restaurant.

And then one day I got the word: My friend had resigned his position to open his own restaurant. He was finally pursuing his dream. Unfortunately, his business did not do as well as he had planned, and after much pain and loss he was forced to watch his dream die.

Many people would look back and say he should never have sacrificed the security of a good job for a risky venture, but I would have to disagree with them. My friend's dream was to one day open his own restaurant, and he achieved his dream. Despite the pain of knowing it didn't succeed as he had hoped, at least he will not as an old man have to face the more crippling pain of knowing that he never even tried to reach his dream. Far happier is the person who has tried and failed than the one who has never even tried. Pursue your dream lest you be haunted by regrets.

RISKS AND REWARDS

Owning your own business can be one of the most challenging and rewarding endeavors you can ever attempt; however, it is not for everyone. There are both risks and sacrifices which accompany self-owned businesses. While still in graduate school, I was able to become a part owner of the furniture business in which I was working. We saw the business grow and additional stores open after we purchased the company from the previous owners. It helped greatly to support my wife and myself as I finished my university training.

I learned many lessons through not only my own experiences but also those of my friends and acquaintances. Let me share five cautions with those of you who may be considering the launching of your own business.

1. Plan to work long, hard hours in the early days of your endeavor. Some entrepreneurs have stated that you don't really own the business, but rather it owns you. There is much truth to this statement. Plan to invest more time than you planned as the business begins. In the beginning, there will be a nonstop string of unusual demands on your time. It has also been stated that one of the advantages of owning your own business is being able to choose to work only half-days—either the first 12 hours or the second 12 hours!

2. Be prepared for additional demands on your wallet. No matter how well you calculate your cost of start-up, there will always be surprises which will drain your finances. One of the major reasons new businesses fail is that they are undercapitalized, and therefore unprepared to withstand the early days when new businesses invariably lose money. Be prepared to lose money on your venture for the entire first year. Unless you are a rarity, you will experience this loss and should be prepared to ride it out.

3. Listen to the advice of those who have gone before you. Listen to their negative comments as well as their encouragements. By drawing on their experiences, you

may be able to keep from repeating some of the mistakes they have made. Don't become so blinded by your optimism that you ignore the facts. The facts are your friends even if they are not what you wanted to see. If you plan to enter the world of business be a realist.

4. Beware of partnerships. They can offer a sense of security and shared responsibility, but they can also lead to major stress if not properly conceived. This is especially true of partnerships with unbelievers. The Bible warns us to avoid becoming unequally yoked with unbelievers. This applies to business as well as to marriage. Both are yokes to be carefully examined in advance.

5. Beware of questionable shortcuts. Not too long ago the world of finance was shocked by the fall of some of its brightest young stars. Michael Milken posted bail of 100 million dollars as he faced charges of fraud in his sale of over a billion dollars in junk bonds. This rising young superstar of the financial world was later convicted and shipped off to prison because of the shady shortcuts he had used in his rise to the top.

The tabloids had a field day as they followed the marital and financial woes of onetime billionaire Donald Trump. His rise to the top of the financial world had been meteoric, or so it seemed. He had taken shortcuts which, though legal, would haunt him later as the world of real estate began to soften. He ended up paying a steep price for taking an unwise shortcut.

SKIPPING RUNGS

Regardless of your chosen field, be cautious of trying to skip rungs on the ladder of success. You may end up missing valuable lessons which could have prepared you to better cope with the demands and pressures of your target position.

A friend of mine had always wanted to pastor a large church. After graduation from seminary he accepted a call to a small church, and immediately the church began to grow and promise a great future. That dream was interrupted when a church of greater size convinced my friend to become their pastor. Thereafter a pattern emerged: My friend in his quest to pastor a large church repeatedly left his present church to accept a larger one. But in so doing he missed some very valuable rungs on the ladder, and when he got his chance at a large church, he discovered that he had no idea what to do. It wasn't long before he was to start a pattern of "trading down" as he went from one church to the next.

As I prepared to enter the ministry, I studied successful evangelical churches and pastors. I discovered that in most cases men have built large and dynamic churches by taking a small church and growing up with it. They have grown at the same pace as the church. This has been true in my own life and ministry. Our church has grown over the ten years I have been here from a church ministering to hundreds to a church ministering to thousands. I have gone through all of the steps with it and have learned valuable lessons that I would have missed had I come in cold.

In my early days at the church, I received an opportunity to candidate at a much larger and better-known ministry. This would have allowed me to skip the struggles for staff and facilities which a growing church faces. I could have stepped in where the work had already been done. Although it was tempting, I said no because I felt there were lessons I would learn in the pain of growing that I might miss and thereby lessen my effectiveness. If I was unable to build a large church, I didn't believe I would be either prepared or deserving to pastor one built by someone else.

THE BEST WAY TO THE TOP

This same principle holds true in every field of endeavor. The best way to the top of the ladder of success is one rung at a time. I have known people whom I call "ladder jumpers." As they climb the company ladder, they spot an opportunity to jump to another company's ladder, but at a couple of rungs higher. Intrigued by the opportunity for rapid advancement, they jump. This pattern may be repeated several times as they continue to jump to different ladders and begin to approach the top.

Unfortunately, many of these people discover that they are the weaker because of the rungs they skipped. Their knowledge of the company and the industry is not as deep as the person who touched all the rungs. There are times when a blockage ahead of you on the company ladder makes switching companies a necessary and wise move, but if done with only an eye for rapid personal advancement, such a move may do more harm than good. Company loyalty is still a characteristic which wise employers weigh carefully when deciding promotions. Find a company you believe in, and then give them a reason to believe in you. Don't be constantly lured into making changes by the promise of greener grass.

Do They Really Need You?

Stress can result when the boss begins to believe that the company can function just as well without you. If he and your co-workers develop questions about whether they really need you, you will feel stress. Once you have a job, make yourself indispensable by learning everything there is to know about the job and the business. Learn what others do and be available to lend support when needed. Learn what your boss does, and then volunteer to help. Learn to do the difficult jobs that no one else wants to do.

Make sure to always be on time. A man who once worked for me was chronically late for meetings and appointments. I am a punctual person, and I hate to waste time waiting for someone else, especially when it happens more than once. One day I sat this worker down and pointed out to him that whenever he entered a room, his first statement was always an apology for being late. He was in marketing, and I pointed out to him that a sales call is greatly weakened when the salesman begins his presentation with an apology for being late! It shows an insensitivity and disrespect for the person forced to wait for you. Be the type of worker whom the boss can count on to be on time.

The same applies to telling the truth. If you make it a practice never to deceive or mislead your boss or fellow workers, you will be held in high regard. Even if telling the whole truth will cause you personal loss, do it anyway rather than risk a damaged reputation because of dishonesty.

One aspect of honesty involves doing what you say you will do. If you commit to get a project done, get it done. This sounds so simple, yet it is an area of weakness with many workers. They may eventually get the job done, but not when they said they would. Or they may get it done only after reminders and pressure from their boss. Still others may eventually get the job done, but with only a half-hearted effort and with poor quality. In all of the above, a boss true to the expectations of his position will bring stress into the life of that employee.

Precious are those workers who, when given an assignment, will 1) get it done on time, 2) get it done without being prodded, and 3) get it done with excellence and enthusiasm. Management will go out of its way to keep such workers happy on the job. Become an indispensable worker, and watch on-the-job stress decline in your life.

WHAT IS YOUR ATTITUDE?

One day while reflecting back upon people I know who have been fired from different jobs in diverse industries, it struck me that the most common reason the majority of them lost their jobs was related to their attitude. While working with salespeople in the furniture business I observed that if their attitude was positive and supportive, every effort was made to keep them employed even if their production was not what it should have been. On the other hand, good salespeople were sometimes released if their attitude had a negative impact on those around them.

In most industries, people with poor *performance* last a lot longer than people with poor *attitudes*. We are told in Ephesians 6:7 to work for our employers "with good will doing service." Keep your attitude positive, and you will face far less stress on the job. Some workers are their own worst enemies in this area.

People see you as you see yourself. If you see yourself as successful and attractive, others will have a similar impression of you. If, on the other hand, you don't like yourself and don't have confidence in yourself, neither will others.

This is clearly illustrated by "Miss Piggy. " This character, created by the late Jim Henson, is viewed as a real "looker" and glamorous. She is the idol of other women because of her beauty, and yet in reality she is just a pig! Although her physical attributes are limited at best, because she believes she is attractive, others see her the same way.

I have seen this phenomenon repeated in real life by people who have nothing to cause them to stand out in a crowd other than a deep belief in themselves. Their confidence is contagious, and those around them view them as attractive, smart, and confident. Conversely, there are others who have much more going for them by way of looks and intelligence, yet because they don't believe in themselves others don't either. Remember, other people will share the attitude you have toward yourself.

HOW TO BE VALUABLE

There are several steps you can take toward presenting a positive and valuable attitude on the job. You can begin by avoiding criticism. When you hear people criticize the boss or other workers to you, you can almost count on the fact that they will criticize *you* when your back is turned. You will save yourself much grief if you make it a policy to avoid criticizing anyone at work, and especially the boss.

Avoid getting embroiled in petty arguments at work. Don't allow co-workers to force you to take a side in disagreements which are nothing more than cheap office politics. Learn to rise above the petty.

Nobody really appreciates a pessimist. There are some workers who feel it is their job to make negative comments about every endeavor anyone attempts. They are especially quick to attack anything that might be new and innovative. These are the people who never rise far in an organization; they get lodged in the middle and cause everyone else discomfort. Pessimists make poor leaders. People beginning a great undertaking want to be encouraged about its possible success rather than be told everything that might go wrong along the way.

Some workers are considered to have an attitude problem because of their inflexibility. They are fine as long as no one breaches the status quo, yet they get thrown into a tizzy when things change. This is unfortunate, because one of the hallmarks of successful companies is their commitment to constant and rapid change. They must be quick to respond to changing markets and trends. Even change implemented too slowly may result in losses.

An inflexible attitude will do a worker harm. Don't be afraid to march into new and untested waters. Resistance may make you look like the enemy.

Employers favor employees who radiate an attitude of control, and don't panic when crisis strikes. Learn to view crisis as opportunity in disguise, a chance to show what you can do when others run and hide. One of my favorite fictional characters has always been James Bond. He portrays the epitome of control under pressure. He lives by the principle that you never let the enemy see you sweat.

My management style is to find the best workers there are, get them pointed in the right direction, and then stay out of their way. Those on my staff who are self-starters love this type of management and excel in their program development. They love the freedom they are given to be creative.

Those who have difficulty with self-direction, however, find this type of leadership very threatening. They would much rather have me looking over their shoulder and telling them what to do next than to figure it out themselves. They lack the attitude of a self-starter. Those who have learned the attitude of self-starting know that employers cherish such workers. Rather than waiting to be told what to do, they just do it.

THE ONLY CHRISTIAN?

I'm thankful for the time I spent in the business world before going into full-time Christian service. I was able to get a taste of what it is like to live a consistent testimony in a complex and competitive world. There were times when I found myself in situations where I was the only person sober or the only one remaining true to his spouse. I learned many lessons which I wish every pastor could learn. I learned that there is a lot of pressure on Christians in the real world, and that to take a clear stand for Jesus is not easy and will not go unnoticed. I learned that I could be a close friend to my unsaved coworkers, but that I could never be "one of the guys" in life-style and in attitude.

Often I found that I was the only Christian working in a particular setting. This put me under tremendous pressure to properly represent Jesus Christ to my co-workers. I might be the only true Christian with whom some of them would ever work, so I had better not give them a distorted picture of Christ.

What an opportunity to show your coworkers the best of Christianity—to show them that Christians can be the best of all workers because we are doing it for Christ! We can do this by being honest, dependable, hard-working, compassionate, forgiving, moral, sober, and exhibiting all the other strengths of character that God wants us to have.

A Christian can do great harm to the cause of Christ if he allows himself to be "one of the boys" in certain areas. Your coworkers are watching to see if you are any different than they are. They want to see if you steal from the company, call in sick when you're not, bad-mouth the boss, gossip about other workers, take long lunch hours, chase women, lie to save your skin, come in late and leave early, plus any number of other office misdemeanors. If you do, you are slandering the reputation of Jesus Christ.

You may be the only living, breathing Christian some of your co-workers will ever encounter. They will formulate their image of Christ by watching your every move. Take care not to give them a distorted view of your Lord!

9

. . . .

STRESSED-OUT CHECKBOOKS

Will Rogers understood the strange lure of money when he said, "Too many people spend money they don't have to buy things they don't want to impress people they don't like." But the special lure of money began long before Rogers penned those words. Two thousand years ago the apostle Paul wrote to the Church in Ephesus that "the love of money is a root of all kinds of evil" (1 Timothy 6:10). This strange love of money continues to haunt men and women to this day. It can cause the nicest of people to do all kinds of evil deeds.

Several years ago the IRS received 300 dollars in currency attached to an anonymous note which read, "Some time ago I cheated on my income tax return, and I haven't had a good night's sleep since then. My hope is that now that I have sent this money I can sleep. P.S. If I still can't sleep, I'll send the rest."

WHAT CAN MONEY BUY?

Our society places so much emphasis on what money *can* buy that we lose sight of what money *cannot* buy. As Paul Tan puts it so well in his *Illustrations*:

Money can buy:

> A bed but not sleep
> Books but not brains
> Food but not appetite
> Finery but not beauty
> A house but not a home
> Medicine but not health
> Luxuries but not culture
> Amusements but not happiness

A crucifix but not a Savior
A church pew but not heaven

When crisis strikes, people begin to evaluate what is important and what is not. It was reported that 11 millionaires went to the bottom of the North Atlantic Ocean after the *Titanic* struck an iceberg that fateful night. As people struggled to get to lifeboats, money was the last thing on their minds. Major A. H. Peuchen left 300,000 dollars in money, jewelry, and securities in a box in his cabin. "The money seemed a mockery at that time," he said later. "I picked up three oranges instead."

MONEY OUT OF CONTROL

The Bible is filled with stories of awful deeds committed by people placing the love of money over the love of people. Joseph was sold by his brothers for 20 pieces of silver (Genesis 37). The sons of Samuel cheated on their responsibilities to God and the temple when they accepted bribes (1 Samuel 8). The love of money caused the rich young ruler to reject Christ (Mark 10). Simon the sorcerer thought he could buy the power of the Holy Spirit with his money (Acts 8). Delilah betrayed Samson for the money she was offered (Judges 16). Ananias and Sapphira loved money so much that they were willing to cheat God (Acts 5). And of course there is the heinous crime of Judas Iscariot, who sold the Son of God for 30 pieces of silver.

The love of money continues to be a major root of all evil. It is one of the primary causes in 85 percent of all divorces. It triggers as many arguments in the home as any other topic. It causes churches to fight and pastors to leave. Its pursuit has caused many a Christian to grow cold toward God as he or she pursues the false god of money.

Money can become a source of tremendous stress in the lives of Christians. Whether people do not have enough to pay their bills, or make it their god, or simply use it improperly, money can bring about stress that is unrelenting and especially cruel. Fortunately, God has given us instructions on how to use our resources without driving ourselves over the edge with stress.

THE TEMPLE THIEVES

Jesus pointed out His displeasure with the love of money when He went nose-to-nose with the money-changers in the temple in Jerusalem. As Matthew records the story in chapter 21,

Jesus had entered Jerusalem just days before He was to be crucified. He electrified the crowds as He healed with a power never seen before. Listen to how the crowd reacted as He made His Triumphal Entry: "A very great multitude spread their garments on the road; others cut down branches from the trees and spread them on the road. Then the multitudes who went before and those who followed cried out, saying: 'Hosanna to the Son of David! Blessed is He who comes in the name of the Lord! Hosanna in the highest!' And when He had come into Jerusalem, all the city was moved, saying, 'Who is this?' So the multitudes said, 'This is Jesus, the prophet from Nazareth of Galilee'" (Matthew 21:8–11).

Followed by this mob of cheering citizens, Jesus stormed into the courtyard of the temple. Because it was the season of Passover, there may have been several hundred thousand people jammed into the temple courtyard. Note what Jesus did first upon entering the temple compound: He went after those who were extorting money from the pilgrims who had come to sacrifice at the temple. We read in Matthew 21:12,13: "Then Jesus went into the temple of God and drove out all those who bought and sold in the temple, and overturned the tables of the moneychangers and the seats of those who sold doves. And He said to them, 'It is written, My house shall be called a house of prayer, but you have made it a den of thieves.'"

These vendors had made a deal with the temple priests. When a pilgrim brought an animal to be sacrificed, the priest would inform him that the animal wasn't pure enough, and to ensure a pure sacrifice he must buy one at an inflated price from the temple sellers. In turn, the sellers would offer the pilgrim a ridiculously low amount to take the "impure" animal off his hands. They would then sell him a "pure" animal for a ridiculously high amount. In more cases than not, it was merely an animal they had taken off the hands of a previously frustrated pilgrim. What a scam! The people hated it, but they had no way to do anything about it.

The money-changers were no better. As each pilgrim arrived to pay his annual "temple tax" he would be told he had the wrong type of currency, and that to rectify this situation he would have to visit one of the temple money-changers. Needless to say, their rates were nothing short of outrageous. And also needless to say, the temple priests shared the kickbacks from the money-changers.

Fully aware of their wicked extortion hidden behind the cover of the temple, Jesus took the gloves off as He entered the courtyard where they sold their wares. How dare they do this to the house of God? They had turned it into a den of thieves.

So much for *their* problem. Now let's turn our attention to how money can cause *us* to miss God's best for *our* lives, and how we can outsmart stress in our finances.

CAUTION: STRESS AT WORK

We all know the stress that can result when there are bills to be paid but no money with which to pay them. There just seems to be too much month at the end of the money! Despite repeated efforts to curtail spending and increase revenues, we find ourselves much like the federal government: drifting deeper and deeper into debt. The credit cards are already maxed out, and another "debt-consolidation loan" is out of the question. Both cars and most of the major appliances need to be repaired or replaced. The kids just keep asking for more money as they grow older, and increasingly money has become the main source of stress in our home. Is there a way of escape before we strike bottom?

Let me share some guidelines that God has given us on how to use what money we possess. If followed, they will not only keep us out of overwhelming debt, but will also help those already buried in debt to begin the long climb out.

As we begin, remember that how you handle your money will both reflect and affect your spiritual walk. People get into trouble with their finances because they fail, either out of ignorance or outright disobedience, to follow God's instructions on the use of their money. Now let's consider the most important principles in money management.

WHOSE MONEY IS IT?

I once had the opportunity to serve as the trustee for the estate of a woman whose husband had passed away leaving a fairly large and complex estate. As trustee, I had the responsibility to oversee the care of her property and money. She was a generous woman and enjoyed giving special gifts to both charities and individuals. As trustee, I was often the one who would deliver a check to one of the unsuspecting charities. They grew to love it every time they saw me pull into their parking lot, and it made me feel like a hero.

I remember one occasion when I met with this generous woman and recommended that she slow down her gift-giving lest she deplete the funds in the trust. Without hesitation she reminded me that all the funds in the trust belonged to her, and that if she chose to give them all away, they were hers to give. After hearing her out, I felt awkward that I had acted stingy with money that wasn't even mine. I realized that I had started to act as if the money in the trust were mine, when in fact it was someone else's. I was merely the trustee, or to use another word, I was the *steward* of the riches of another person.

This is the first step for the Christian to get his financial house in order: to recognize that all he seems to possess is in reality God's. We as Christians are simply to serve as trustees or stewards of His wealth while we are on this earth. We must be careful to avoid being either greedy or careless with the assets He has entrusted to our care.

With this in mind, giving to the work of the Lord must take priority over spending on ourselves. After all, we are returning to God only a small portion of what is His in the first place.

Of all the verses which give instructions on how to support the Lord's work, I like the way it is summed up in 1 Corinthians 16:1,2: "Now concerning the collection for the saints, as I have given orders to the churches of Galatia, so you must do also: On the first day of the week let each one of you lay something aside, storing up as he may prosper, that there be no collections when I come." The apostle Paul was sharing with the church in Corinth four principles on how to give to the work of the Lord. He added that these were not unique to them but were also given to the churches of Galatia. These same principles apply to believers in churches around the world and across the ages.

FOUR VITAL PRINCIPLES

1. "On the first day of the week let each one of you lay something aside." Giving should be regular and systematic. The early Christians were instructed to do it on the first day of the week, which is Sunday. By doing it regularly, they were reminded at the start of each new week of God's provision in their lives. They received the opportunity weekly to thank God for meeting their needs as they gave back a portion to God.

This method also allowed them to give a little extra if God had blessed them with extra during the past week.

2. We are to bring our gifts *to the local church* as we gather to meet on the first day of the week. The leaders of the local church will then discern where the combined gifts can best be invested in the needs of the Lord's work.

   This is called "storehouse giving," and is seen in other places in the Bible. In Acts 4:33–37 we see the example of Barnabas who, after selling a piece of land, brought the money and laid it at the apostles' feet. They in turn determined how it should be distributed in the work of the Lord.

   One of the advantages of storehouse giving is that combined giving allows churches to send missionaries to the field, whereas by themselves the giving of most individuals would fall far short of what is needed. This combined giving also allows churches to provide buildings and support ministries to care for the needs of the local congregation.

   A second advantage arises from the fact that the church leaders who make decisions about the distribution of the funds have been called by God to serve, and have been confirmed in their ministry by the entire congregation. They should be godly men in charge of God's money. They should also possess a view of the entire congregation and its needs, and be able to make decisions based on their overview of the entire ministry.

   There is nothing wrong with believers giving gifts ddirectly to individuals in the ministry or to parachurch organizations. Many of these are doing a great work for the Lord. But this should be over and above your giving to the local church. Your first responsibility is to the local church rather than to some far-flung television ministry. Although you may have little knowledge of how that faraway ministry is using your gifts, your local church leaders are under the close scrutiny of the local congregation, which is able to see that their gifts are used as intended.

3. First Corinthians 16:2 states, "Let *each one of you* lay something aside." Each believer is instructed to give to the work of the Lord regardless of how much or how

little he possesses. The key is *total involvement by all the people* and not just by a limited group.

Each is to give "as he may prosper." Different people have received different financial blessings from God, and this will be reflected in their ability to give, but all must commit to give something.

4. Each believer is instructed to give *"as he may prosper,"* which implies that we are to see equal sacrifice, not equal giving. For some people, giving 10 percent is the ultimate sacrifice, whereas for others 10 percent may just be pocket change. The key is for *all God's people to give sacrificially,* or until it hurts to give.

Many Christians who are experiencing stress in their finances have fallen short in the area of stewardship. They have not yet settled the question of whose money it is—theirs or God's. They are waiting until they have enough extra before they start to give to the work of the Lord, and yet they never seem to have enough. They have somehow gotten things backward, and consequently are experiencing much unnecessary financial stress.

Luke 6:38 challenges us, "Give and it will be given to you: good measure, pressed down, shaken together, and running over will be put into your bosom. For with the same measure that you use, it will be measured back to you." That's God's Word on the matter: Give and it shall be given to you, whether meagerly or in abundance—the choice is yours.

SAVE OR SPEND?

Surveys show that when it comes to saving money, Americans receive poor marks. We are a society which has turned spending money into an art form, while saving money is something that occurs less and less each decade.

The creation of the Social Security Administration in response to the tragedy of the Great Depression of the 1930s has caused many Americans to focus on the present with little concern for their retirement years. They have fallen prey to the misconception that Social Security is a retirement program, whereas in reality it was designed to be "survival insurance" for those who had nothing else or who needed to supplement their pension or retirement savings. It was never designed to be a total personal retirement program. This is evidenced by the fact that the average

Social Security recipient today receives 550 dollars per month—
hardly enough to provide for those "Golden Years" of retirement!

Americans have so focused on gratifying their present needs
that few people give serious thought to preparing for their future
needs, and many end up unprepared for current emergencies or
future survival. They feel stress in their lives because they have
failed to provide a cushion to protect themselves from those
unexpected falls which are so common.

THE THREE-PRONGED PLAN

To reduce stress in your financial world, develop a three-
pronged plan for your savings. These three levels should
include savings for 1) emergencies, 2) major purchases, and 3)
retirement.

1. *Emergencies.* Financial consultants advise setting aside
   enough money to carry you through a period of three
   months with no income. Although no one plans on being
   out of work, we all know that unemployment does
   happen in the lives of people constantly.

   This fund should be made priority number one in
   your financial planning. It will not be easy to establish
   and will require both discipline and a plan, but once in
   place, it will afford you much security and far less fear of
   the unexpected.

   Just prior to my sitting down to write this chapter, my
   wife informed me that she thinks the transmission is
   going out in our van. Only minutes before this I had
   noticed a fresh oil slick under my car, and as I walked
   through the garage on the way into the house I noticed
   water dripping out the bottom of our hot-water heater. I
   suspect if the truth were known, there are several other
   appliances in our household which will quit working
   this next year. These are the kinds of unexpected expenses
   which can cause great stress in a marriage if the partners
   vent their financial frustrations on each other.

   The pain of the unexpected can be greatly reduced
   once you understand that due to their mechanical nature,
   appliances and automobiles will inevitably break down.
   You should expect this to happen and plan for it in your
   emergency savings fund. Accept it as a cost of living and
   don't allow it to ruin your day.

2. *Major purchases.* An epidemic of borrowing has swept across America. Young couples begin their lives together by going into debt to purchase major items and then spend decades struggling to get out from under their debt. Every time they turn around they are bombarded with advertising instructing them to "buy now, pay later." As their indebtedness increases, they end up paying a major portion of their income to cover the interest they owe on their debts. If this interest could be funneled into saving, their lives would be much more secure and stress-free.

The key to avoiding the above scenario is to learn to save up for major purchases and pay cash for them. Buy things "the old-fashioned way"—pay cash for them rather than hoping you get them paid off before they wear out. Discipline yourself to faithfully save money for major purchases.

I personally would include automobile purchases in this category. Too many people are slaves to multiple car payments. They never really get a car paid off before it is worn out, and then they incur an even larger monthly cost for its replacement. If they could ever get far enough ahead to pay for a car up front, they could probably continue to be free of car payments. My adherence to this plan has often meant driving cars longer than most people while saving for a replacement vehicle, but the pain is minimized by the fact that the car is paid for.

3. *Retirement.* The third form of savings involves long-term preparation for that time when you retire and will no longer receive your present income. Almost anyone can make adequate preparation for retirement if he or she is systematic and begins early in life. The key is to *develop a plan and then stick to it.* As has often been stated, "People don't plan to fail . . . they merely fail to plan."

Whether through your company's retirement program or a plan of your own, get involved in a program that automatically puts a portion of your salary toward a safe retirement fund. Especially helpful are those programs which take the money out of your regular paycheck. Although you may miss the money for the first couple of months, after awhile you will no longer even consider it as income, and all the while it will be going toward your retirement. Actually, the amount you invest is less important than the fact that it is invested each and every month. A successful retirement strategy has to be systematic to work effectively.

The second key to developing a successful retirement plan is to start early. When such a program is begun early, time becomes the investor's ally, whereas later in life time becomes the investor's enemy. Most financial planners agree that people must get serious about preparing for retirement by the age of 40. After that time, substantial sacrifices will have to be made to ensure a comfortable retirement.

If you will discipline yourself to systematically save at a young age, you will be astonished at how the laws of compounded interest will work in your favor. For example, the "Rule of 72" is the basic equation used to figure out how long it will take for your investment to double in value at any given interest rate. Merely divide the number 72 by the interest rate of your investment, and the resulting number will be the number of years it will take for that investment to double in value because of the compounding interest. For example, at 9 percent a 2000-dollar investment will double in value in eight years (72 divided by 9 equals 8).

To realize the power of this equation, assume that the 2000 dollars was invested by a young man at age 20 and allowed to earn 9 percent until he retired at age 68. By that time his 2000 dollars will double in value six times and be worth 128,000 dollars. And that is without ever investing another cent in the account!

If this same young man had waited until he was 28 to invest his 2000 dollars at 9 percent, he would have seen his investment double five times and be worth only half as much, or 64,000 dollars, at age 68. Needless to say, time is the ally of the young when it comes to preparing for retirement. Unfortunately, retirement is usually the least concern for most people in their twenties. However, for those with enough foresight, it is the best time to begin.

How Much Are You Spending?

Many Christian families struggle because they have not disciplined themselves to save systematically. Some of them counter by saying that their finances are so tight that there is literally not an extra dime left at the end of the month to put toward savings. Put simply, the key to making ends meet in your finances is to spend less each month than you make. This applies to the person squeaking by on 15,000 dollars per year as well as to the individual making 150,000 dollars per year. The key for both is to spend less than they make. Either of them can get into deep financial straits by spending more than they make, regardless of whether the amount is 15,000 or 150,000 dollars per year.

It is never too soon to develop a realistic budget to regulate your spending. Some people receive a rude awakening when they prepare a truly accurate budget. To their shock, they realize the reason they never seem to have any money is that their monthly obligations, coupled with their other expenditures, exceed their income. The problem is most likely tied to their spending habits.

Many people have difficulty sensing the difference between things they *want* and things they actually *need*. If they would take a minute to think, they would realize that although they may *want* that new set of golf clubs, they do not *need* them. If they want them and can afford to pay for the clubs, there is nothing wrong with buying them. However, if they are already struggling with debts and bills, each purchase must be analyzed to determine whether it is a "want" or a "need."

Many times we get interested in something because a friend of ours has just purchased one. I saw this happen in a church we attended when one family had a swimming pool installed. Soon several other families had their backyards torn up as swimming pools were being installed. The same is true with new cars. It can be like a virus as people fall victim to the "new-car fever" they may have caught while riding in their best friend's new chariot. Don't let impulse buying destroy your carefully designed budget. Learn to discern between "wants" and "needs."

TWELVE CRUCIAL QUESTIONS

In an attempt to help people determine whether they are chronic overspenders *Money* magazine asked 15 credit counselors and financial planners to draw up the following checklist. People were asked to answer either true or false to each of the following twelve statements.

1. You spend money on the expectation that your income will rise.
2. You take cash advances on one credit card to pay off another.
3. You spend over 20 percent of your income on credit-card bills.
4. You often fail to keep an accurate record of your purchases.
5. You have applied for more than three cards in the past year.
6. You regularly pay for groceries with a credit card because you need to.
7. You often hide your credit-card purchases from your family.
8. Owning several credit cards makes you feel richer.
9. You pay off your monthly credit-card bills but let others slide.
10. You like to collect cash from friends in restaurants, then charge the tab on your credit card.
11. You almost always make only the minimum payment on your credit-card bill.
12. You have trouble imagining your life without credit.

The financial advisers concluded that if you had two "true" answers, you must stop your borrowing, draw up a budget, pay off your bills, and reevaluate your spending habits. If you scored more than five "true" answers, you would be wise to consult a financial counselor for help in changing your habits—beginning by destroying your credit cards!

OUT OF THE BLACK HOLE

The natural result of overspending is stifling debt which permeates every aspect of a person's life. Once debt crosses a certain threshold, even sleep deserts the person living in fear of the impending consequences. Of all couples who have divorced, 85 percent cite financial pressures as one of the key reasons for arguments in their homes. The kids are affected too as they see the pressure turn their parents into tense and short-tempered people.

It is easier to stay out of debt than it is to extradite yourself once already in debt. It is a long and steep hill you must climb to get out of stifling debt, but it can be done.

If you are just starting out on your own, you have a tremendous opportunity to avoid falling into the black hole of debt. By heeding the three principles of stewardship, saving, and controlled spending you should be able, apart from very unusual circumstances, to avoid stifling debt. Do these and you won't have to worry about how to get out of debt, because you won't fall into debt in the first place.

Having said this, I am aware that the problem faced by most people is getting out of the black hole of debt in which they are already mired. To be honest, it is difficult to get out of debt. It is not accomplished without a disciplined and well-planned strategy. Here are seven steps advocated by the Stewardship Services Foundation which should help in all but the most difficult situations:

STEP 1: Stop all new indebtedness immediately.

STEP 2: Promise to put all extra income into debt retirement.

STEP 3: Sell all depreciating items for which you are now in debt.
a. Replace with a less expensive item.
b. Get out from under all monthly payments.
c. Sell all items with maintenance and upkeep costs first.

STEP 4: Closely examine food costs. You should be able to make a 15 percent minimum cut.

STEP 5: Begin immediately to "do it yourself" instead of paying for services.

STEP 6: Set a challenging goal for debt retirement on a pay-period basis, and make all the necessary sacrifices until you are out of debt.

STEP 7: Make getting out of debt a family effort. Let every member participate with his own resources.

You are certainly not alone if you are struggling with stifling debt in your life. While preaching in our church on this matter of debt, as soon as I stated that I was about to give "seven steps to getting out of debt," just about every person immediately pulled out pencil and paper to take notes. Don't allow debt to defeat you. You are not alone in your struggle to free yourself from its powerful hold, and with a workable plan it can be done!

10

SATANIC STRESS

With the publication of *This Present Darkness*, Frank Peretti seemed to rekindle the interest of the Christian community in the dark side of life . . . the side inhabited by the devil and his legions of demons. Along with the increased interest came debate over how much each Christian should be concerned with the creatures of the dark side.

The debate is not new. It was discussed years earlier by C. S. Lewis, who finally concluded, "There are two equal and opposite errors into which our race can fall about the devils. One is to disbelieve in their existence. The other is to believe, and to feel an excessive and unhealthy interest in them. They themselves are equally pleased by both errors and hail a materialist or a magician with the same delight."

I couldn't have summed it up better than this well-known quotation by Lewis. We need to avoid the twin pitfalls of either 1) denying the existence of Satan and his demonic host, or 2) becoming preoccupied with things associated with the devil. Although wisdom would mandate a healthy respect for such evil power, Scripture tells us that we have within us a power greater than that possessed by Satan.

Although the power of God is infinitely greater than that of Satan, Christians who are not wary of what Satan is able to do run the risk of opening their lives for his attacks. When Christians allow Satan a toehold in their lives, stress can build to a sinister level. In this chapter we will show how the enemy works to topple Christians into the despair of stress. We will first clearly identify our adversary and describe some of his favorite methods of attack. Then we will show from God's Word the advantage each Christian has at his disposal in the battle for control of his life.

YOU ARE AT WAR!

As the book of Ephesians draws to a close, the apostle Paul issues a stern warning to Christians to be on guard regarding their adversary, the devil: "Finally, my brethren, be strong in the Lord and in the power of His might. Put on the whole armor of God, that you may be able to stand against the wiles of the devil. For we do not wrestle against flesh and blood, but against principalities, against powers, against the rulers of the darkness of this age, against spiritual hosts of wickedness in the heavenly places. Therefore take up the whole armor of God, that you may be able to withstand in the evil day, and having done all, to stand" (Ephesians 6:10-13).

In Ephesians 6 we see the picture of a warrior making preparation to do battle against an awesome adversary. Each Christian is such a warrior, and is required with or without his consent to do battle against his adversary the devil. We can have victory in this struggle, but only if we heed the warnings and instructions given in God's Word.

In verse 10 we are told that we must be strong in the Lord. This is not the type of warfare to enter without the power of God behind us. Put simply, we will be overmatched by the adversary. We must be strong *in the Lord* and let *His* power flow through us. God has provided all the necessary armor to ensure our victory, and we are told to put on the entire armor of God. The armor is available and powerful, but unless we personally strap it on, it is of little value to us.

If a warrior enters a battle improperly armed and protected, he will very likely lose the battle. Here are some mistakes that Christians commonly make regarding their armor.

WHAT IS YOUR ARMOR?

Many Christians are walking in the midst of their enemy without a stitch of armor to protect them. For whatever reason, they have not grasped the magnitude of the danger that their adversary poses. *The armor must be put on by each individual soldier.* I can't strap it on you, and you can't strap it on me; it must be done by each person for himself. Even though there is enough armor available to cover every one of God's children, much of it hangs useless in the armory of God because some of His soldiers have foolishly gone into battle without proper protection.

Our adversary is not only evil, but he is also clever and

experienced. Through the ages he has learned that he cannot pierce the Christian's armor, but that he can find any number of Christians who have neglected to put on one or more of the pieces of armor. It is for this reason that we are instructed to put on the *whole* armor of God and not just selected pieces of it.

A chain is only as strong as its weakest link, and so it is with your armor. Although you may be covered over your whole body with the mighty armor of God, if you have neglected just one piece, that is where Satan will attack you. In a military battle, the general studies the enemy's strengths and weaknesses, and then he attacks at the point of weakest defense.

The armor of God is described in Ephesians 6:14-18. Examine your life to see if you have prudently taken advantage of the *whole* armor of God as described in these verses. If you feel besieged by the enemy in a particular area of your life, it may be that you have neglected that area of protection in your suit of armor and that Satan has discovered your vulnerability.

DON'T WAIT TILL TOO LATE

Seatbelts and shoulder straps are wonderful safety features which can greatly reduce the risk of death or serious injury to people in an automobile accident. But each year thousands die or suffer serious injury because they were not wearing their seatbelts. Those fortunate enough to survive a trip through the windshield of their car would agree that if they had it to do over again, they would have used the safety equipment to protect themselves. Unfortunately, it is too late to put it on after the accident has occurred, for the damage has already been done.

The same can be said about the safety equipment provided free of charge for each Christian. It is sufficient to protect from harm, but only if it is put on prior to the point of attack. The enemy can strike so fast that there is insufficient time to struggle into the armor once the battle has begun. To be most effective, the armor has to be in place prior to satanic attack. Just as soldiers are cautious to have every piece of armor properly placed prior to the enemy's attack, so we as Christians must be ready before we feel the heat of the enemy's approach.

Surprise can be one of the most effective means of attacking a superior foe. The attacker may wait patiently for months for a window of opportunity in which his targets become complacent and relax their defenses. To be most effective, the aggressor will strike when it is least expected. Although his targets may possess vastly superior armor and weapons, they may suffer tremendous loss because they got caught by a surprise attack.

We stand daily under the watchful scrutiny of a wicked and brilliant strategist whose avowed aim is to destroy us. Satan is experienced enough to know that most Christians will grow relaxed and complacent over a period of time. He knows that to attack when the full armor is in place is to invite defeat, but to strike an unprepared Christian can lead to victory . . . and so he waits. We need to keep the armor on at all times!

By definition an accident is a surprise, since it strikes when least expected. So it is with satanic attack. It would be much easier to combat if we knew the moment of his attack, but the devil is much too wily to give us that advantage.

KNOW YOUR ENEMY

Many a nation has suffered greatly because they underestimated either the power or the resolve of their adversary. In the 1930s the nations of the world watched as Adolf Hitler began to re-arm the Third Reich, but they failed to honestly assess how powerful his forces had become. It was only after the Second World War was fully raging that the rest of the world understood the magnitude of the adversary's power and resolve.

The world of boxing was shocked in 1990 when they watched as a relative unknown by the name of Buster Douglas defeated Iron Mike Tyson, the man they said was unbeatable. Tyson made the terrible mistake of underestimating his enemy, and he lost his crown because of it.

Many Christians have lost potential crowns in glory because they underestimated their adversary the devil. Satan would love for us to believe he is a mischievous little guy with a pitchfork and long pointed tail, but unfortunately he possesses vast strength and an invincible army. He is the most powerful of God's created beings.

Michael is called the "archangel of God," and as such he possesses incredible power, yet in Jude 9 we read, "Michael the archangel, in contending with the devil, when he disputed about the body of Moses, dared not bring against him a reviling accusation." If Michael the archangel must use caution in his dealings with the devil, we are foolish to take him lightly.

SATAN'S EMPIRE

Satan's power is seen in the vast empire over which he rules. Ephesians 6:12 gives us a brief peek at the structure of his empire: "We do not wrestle against flesh and blood, but against principalities, against powers, against the rulers of the darkness of this age, against spiritual hosts of wickedness in the heavenly places." We are warned that we are up against an enemy with more than human power.

In Revelation 12:3,4 we see an intimation that when Lucifer sinned against God, as many as one-third of the angels of heaven followed him in his wicked attempt to become God. They were cast out of heaven with him.

Today these fallen angels are more commonly referred to as demons. They possess unusual powers as well as the resolve to bring as many humans as possible to hell with them. Like any well-organized army, they have different assignments and areas of strength, and like the angels of heaven, they have differing levels of leadership. These leaders are named by title in Ephesians 6:12, and include the following:

1. *Principalities.* Called the *archas* in Greek, these are the "arch-demons" or Satan's heavy hitters. They are the generals who have the responsibility of leading the other demons in their attacks.

2. *Powers.* Called *exousia* in the Greek, these are the elite warriors in the army of Lucifer. Whereas the "principalities" specialize in directing the demons, the "powers" are the demons who are called upon to fight when mighty warriors are needed. They are the ones assigned to bring down the mighty men of God who have the gifts to reach the world for Christ. As Satan's elite corps, their job is to destroy the men and women who are leading in the cause of Christ on the earth.

3. *Rulers of the darkness of this age.* Called *cosmokratorias* in the Greek, these are the demons assigned to influence the leaders of our world to do evil. They are the invisible powers behind not only men such as Adolf Hitler and Saddam Hussein, but also those who do not seem to be so evil. Their responsibility is to influence world leaders on all levels to use their power to stymie the plan of God for this world.

In Daniel 10:12,13 we hear the testimony of an angel who had been assigned to help the King of Persia ward off one of these powerful agents of Satan: "He said to me, 'Do not fear, Daniel, for from the day that you set your heart to understand, and to humble yourself before your God, your words were heard; and I have come because of your words. But the prince of the kingdom of Persia withstood me twenty-one days; and behold, Michael, one of the chief princes, came to help me, for I had been left alone there with the kings of Persia.'"

In these verses we have a picture of mighty satanic demons doing battle with one of God's loyal angels in a realm unseen by human eyes. The battle centered around the leaders of Persia, which is modern-day Iran, as it was to be used as God's tool in the unfolding of prophecy. Daniel was in Babylon, which is modern-day Iraq, as it too was part of God's unfolding prophetic plan. Satan had sent the big boys in an attempt to thwart God's plan. After the battle had raged for 21 days, Michael the archangel burst into Persia and the battle was quickly won by the angels of God.

4. *Spiritual hosts of wickedness in heavenly places.* Called *pneumatik* in the Greek, these fallen angels appear to surround our world and work daily to advance the cause of Satan. They are at his beck and call to do whatever is necessary to bring glory and honor to their leader, Satan, by keeping the unsaved away from Jesus Christ, and by causing Christians to stumble in their walk with Christ. They appear sufficient in number to allow at least one to be assigned to every man, woman, and child on this earth. You can be assured that those assigned to ruin the testimony of Christians are especially bright and take great pleasure when they succeed in their heinous vocation.

We receive an image from these words of an evil host so numerous that it forms a dark cloud which hovers over the earth. They are powerful and can't be beaten with a keen intellect, physical might, or well-organized church programs. We have one defense, and that is the armor of God. With that armor properly placed, the Christian can stand against the horrible host

and they must flee. If, on the other hand, the battle breaks out
while the Christian is unarmed, great damage will follow.

PLAN AND COUNTERPLAN

Our enemy possesses not only the power but also the resolve
in the battle for your Christian life. Ephesians 6:11 instructs us to
put on the whole armor of God in order that we may be able to
stand against the *wiles* of the devil. "Wiles" is a translation of the
Greek word *methodeia*, from which we get the word "methodical."
It refers to an attack which is not only powerful, but also
systematic and relentless. The Greek word *methodeia* means "to
follow after a thing systematically, to learn it, to write it down,
and to analyze it."

Just as God has a plan for your life, Satan has an evil
counterplan. He declared war on you the moment you accepted
Jesus Christ as your Lord and Savior. You are now his avowed
enemy, and he will use all his resources and experience to bring
you down. Remember that Satan has many centuries of
experience in learning how to crack supposedly uncrackable
Christians. Don't ever make the mistake of underestimating either
the power or the resolve of your enemy. Periods of apparent
peace are just the lull before the soon-coming storm. Get that
armor on!

Remember the saying, "If you want war, prepare for peace; if
you want peace, prepare for war." This is just as true in the life
of the Christian as it is in the conflicts which arise between nations.
We are daily involved in a war that has been declared upon us
by Satan. That war will rage with or without our consent. It is a
war which must be fought by each and every believer.

DESTROYING THE SOURCE

To defeat an enemy, it is imperative that the source of its
weapons of war be destroyed. In World War Two, Allied
bombing raids were directed at the factories which produced the
weapons used by the enemy to wage war. This same goal led
the United States and its coalition partners to begin the war
against Iraq by targeting the armories and factories which were
used to produce the weapons of war.

A similar strategy is employed by Satan in his efforts to cripple
the cause of Christ. His greatest attacks are aimed at the arsenals
of Christianity: the true churches around the world which are

preparing the soldiers of the cross who will wage unrelenting war against Satan. J. Vernon McGee said it this way: "I do not think the devil is concentrating on the night clubs or on skid row or in the underworld or in the Mafia. I think he is concentrating on the church on Sunday morning. He is working on the spiritual, and too many sleepy Christians seem to be totally unaware of that . . . . The spiritual battle is being fought wherever a man is giving out the Word of God, where a church is standing for the Word of God. That is the place the devil wants to destroy, and that is the place of the spiritual battle."[2]

Satan knows that a mature Christian, fully armed and prepared for battle, is an awesome challenge to his plans and must be stopped prior to maturation. So he uses his wiles to attempt to stunt his growth and reduce his effectiveness for Christ.

THE TACTIC OF DOUBT

When the devil went to work on Eve in the Garden of Eden, he lured her into doubting the Word of God. God had told Adam and Eve they could eat of every tree in the Garden except one, and of course that was the temptation Satan chose to use in his assault.

God had told them they would die if they ate its fruit, so Satan placed the seed of doubt in Eve's mind. Listen to Satan's comments in Genesis 3:4,5: "The serpent said to the woman, 'You will not surely die. For God knows that in the day you eat of it your eyes will be opened, and you will be like God, knowing good and evil.'"

You know the rest of the story: Eve believed the word of the devil instead of the Word of God and convinced her husband to follow suit.

Satan's tactics have changed little since the Garden of Eden; he still attempts to get the children of God to doubt their Father's Word. Instead of the Garden, he does his work inside evangelical churches, Christian colleges, and seminaries. Instead of the serpent, he uses misguided college professors, liberal seminary professors, and unsaved pastors to cause their followers to call God's Word into question. He sows tares in the church, people who strive to become teachers and leaders so they can cause a greater number of Christians to doubt God's Word.

It is important never to lose sight of the fact that Satan is called a liar and the father of liars. As such he can be very convincing. He uses people with all kinds of academic credentials to try to lead others astray. Satan is no fool; he knows that the better his agents appear to the members of the congregation, the more effective they will be in their work of deception. Many times they will be 95 percent correct in their doctrine. Because of the greater credibility this gains them, their 5 percent error is all the more dangerous. Here are three major areas in which Satan and his agents attack God's truth.

1. *God's love.* One of the cardinal doctrines of the faith is that God is love. Any teaching which implies otherwise is incorrect and is designed by Satan to cause doubt. Once a person begins to doubt that God loves him, he has reason to question everything else, from his salvation to God's daily care over his life.

2. *God's power.* Many Christians give God no chance to show His power because they never attempt anything that requires faith. They have placed their trust in their own talents and abilities rather than stepping out in faith and rejoicing in how God provides for their needs.

   I spoke recently with a friend who, despite his own excellent work habits, lost his job and for three months had been unable to find a new one. After he had exhausted every avenue, several men from the church began to pray for God to take care of three major financial hurdles he faced. They even prayed that God would not just give him a job, but the specific job which he really wanted even though his chances of getting it were slim. God loves this kind of challenge and really "showed His stuff." Before three days had gone by, my friend saw each specific prayer answered. What a show of power! And yet it never would have been seen had there not first been a need to rely upon God's power.

   Our church has what we refer to as "God-sized goals." Too many churches are run like corporations and will never attempt something for God unless it can be accomplished with their present resources and income. When they achieve their goals, it is not much different from some corporation meeting its goals. I like "God-sized goals," which can only be reached if God flexes His muscles and shows His power. When that type of goal is reached, everyone can join together in singing, "To *God* be the glory, great things *He* has done."

3.   *God's Word.* Satan's first attack was on the Word of God, and today his favorite target is still the Word of God, the Bible. The Bible contains God's promises to all mankind. If Satan can cause a Christian to doubt whether the Bible can be trusted, he can undermine the foundation of his faith.

When dealing with Christians, Satan is too clever for a frontal assault on the Bible, so he tries to get people to question whether there might be certain parts which contain errors or are not to be taken literally. He always tries to gain a beachhead in his doubt crusade. In the Garden, he didn't question all of what God had said when tempting Eve, but rather picked one area and hit it hard. He continues this tactic today in his attacks on the Bible.

Doubt is the antithesis of faith; the two can't coexist. You must choose to believe God, who is the epitome of truth, or Satan, who is known by his reputation as the father of lies.

DIVIDE AND CONQUER

In battle, wise commanders try to divide their opponents. They try to drive a wedge between the two wings of an advancing army. They attempt to cut through their supply lines and divide them from their base of support. Division will almost always weaken any type of defense.

One of Satan's most effective strategies is to cause division among Christians. He absolutely loves it when his efforts result in Christians attacking fellow Christians rather than trying to reach the lost for Christ. They become bloodied and exhausted from fighting those who should be their allies. Usually the cause of division is not even doctrinal but rather a difference of opinion on worship style or music or something trivial. Satan must enjoy getting such infights started, and then standing back with his demons and chuckling at the foolishness of the brethren.

Can you imagine a war in which you were able to stand back and watch as rival factions of your opponent's army began to shoot each other? A wise commander would wait until they had exhausted each other, and then attack the weakened enemy. That is exactly why Satan promotes division within the body of Christ.

DISTORTING THE TRUTH

We live in a society which has become totally saturated in existentialism. Let me try to define this term as simply as possible: Existentialism declares that there is no absolute truth, but that truth is subjective and may differ for each person. An existentialist proclaims that what is right for him may not be right for others.

This is the philosophical basis behind secular humanism, which states that there are no absolute standards to be upheld. Humanists deny that God has a right to tell mankind what to do, and insist instead that mankind will determine what is right. They subordinate God to the various opinions of mankind.

Even though the dangers of such a philosophy should be obvious, the seeds of existentialism have now sprouted within the Christian church. Pure and unquestioned biblical doctrine has become buried under a pile of human opinions. With cries of "Love unites and doctrine divides," many churches have chosen to seek unity at the expense of doctrinal purity. Many who profess to be Christians are willing to accept as brothers those who fail to recognize even the cardinal doctrines of Christianity.

Others claim that they are Christians in their own special way. They claim that their personal faith is something between them and God, even though it may contradict God's revealed Word. Still others claim that God has given them a personal revelation, despite the fact that it may be directly opposite to what God has revealed in the Bible.

Throughout the centuries the Bible has been the anchor of the Christian faith. It is the unchanging Word of God among a world of changing opinions. When cut adrift from this anchor, the church falls victim to every wind of heresy which may blow. The Bible is the truth of God revealed to mankind, and any attempts to supplant it with the collective opinions of churches, denominations, or theologians are distortions of the truth, and as such are the work of the enemy to cut the church loose from what even Satan himself knows to be true.

In the pieces of our armor as listed in Ephesians 6, it is no coincidence that the first piece to be mentioned is the belt of *truth*. In the picture being drawn of a Roman legionnaire, the belt was foundational to providing the proper armor. While at peace, the soldiers wore baggy tunics which were comfortable but which in battle could trip them while they tried to run or fight. At the outbreak of battle the baggy tunic was pulled up tight and tucked into the belt.

In addition, the belt was used to hold the warrior's other weapons while his hands remained free for combat. Without such a belt, he could easily become entangled during a battle, or lose the fight because he had no place to hold his weapons without using his hands.

Because pure and undistorted truth is foundational for the Christian, it is called the belt in the Christian's armor. Without a clear understanding of what is true and what is a lie, Christians are vulnerable to satanic attacks. Even as Satan continually attempts to distort God's truth, Christians must make it their lifelong pursuit to learn all of God's truth as revealed to mankind in the Bible. Christians must remember that truth is not subjective: People do not determine what is or is not truth; God has already determined that, and has told us to read all about it in the Bible. The truth of God's Word can never be revoked, amended, or overruled by church councils or church leaders. Beware of attempts to distort the Word of God; Satan is behind the movement somewhere!

THE POWER OF DISTRACTION

I have an old garden hose in my backyard which has long since seen its better days. With each passing season it seems to acquire a new set of leaks. Taken individually, each single hole has little impact on the performance of the hose, but when added to the rest of the leaks, so much water is lost before it reaches the nozzle that the hose no longer serves its purpose as a conduit for water. It has acquired too many distractions to allow it to function as it was designed.

Satan discovered long ago that many a fine and dedicated Christian can be rendered ineffective if enough distractions can be brought into his or her life. These distractions don't have to involve activities that are inherently sinful, and in fact Satan knows that seemingly harmless activities are especially effective in distracting Christians from accomplishing God's purpose for their lives.

Some Christians are so involved in the pursuit of recreation, education, athletics, or their job that they have little time or energy left to serve Jesus Christ. They are much like the garden hose: Their time and energy are leaking out in so many different areas that only a trickle is coming out of the nozzle.

Just because an activity is not included in God's list of taboos does not mean it may not be wrong for you. Anything that causes you to become distracted from serving God as He intends is an improper distraction of your energy.

Some Christians believe they are in a 30-year retirement plan. Having served Christ diligently during their youth and as they raised their children, they reach the age of 50 and declare that they have put in their time, and now it is time for the younger couples to "pay their dues." Their time now becomes consumed with lengthy vacations, weekend getaways, or other personal pursuits of pleasure. They forget that the Great Commission applies to every Christian regardless of age and does not contain a retirement provision. It is to be pursued with the same commitment shown by the apostle Paul in 1 Thessalonians 2:8 when he declared, "Affectionately longing for you, we were well pleased to impart to you not only the gospel of God but also our own lives, because you had become dear to us."

THE SLOW SLIDE

Satan enjoys the challenge of tempting Christians to slide almost imperceptibly into sin. Often the drift is so gradual that the person fails even to notice until he or she is far gone. It usually involves adopting the world's life-style and pleasures before accepting its philosophies. Christians become enamored with some of the pleasures that our world has to offer and gradually become so much a part of it that few people can discern that they are even Christians. Romans 12:2 tells us, "Do not be conformed to this world, but be transformed." Satan wants you to live and act like an unsaved person. Beware of his conforming power!

FATAL DABBLING

Satan looks for every possible opportunity to undercut the growth of each Christian. He does this against our will and without our permission. Even when we stand to resist him, he can make life miserable for us. I can't understand why a person would actually invite Satan to come and make his life miserable, and yet that is exactly what many believers do when they dabble in the occult.

Throughout God's Word, we are promised victory over Satan. We are told that greater is He that is in us than he that is in the world. We are told to stand up to Satan, to strap on the whole armor of God and wage battle against him. We are told to resist the devil and he will flee from us.

In war, it is easier to keep an enemy out of a piece of land than to dislodge him once he has gotten entrenched in his defenses. Yet Christians who dabble in things with satanic attachments are allowing just that. It is as if they are saying "Come and get me!" to Satan. It is bad enough when Satan is cleverly disguised in what appears to be a harmless activity and catches Christians by surprise, but it is quite another thing for Christians to dabble in areas with obvious satanic roots. They are inviting disaster and will not be disappointed.

Some of the more obvious invitations to disaster include tarot cards, Ouija boards, seances, and astrology. Not as obviously connected but equally dangerous are movies with satanic themes, some Eastern religions, and many current songs and their videos. Parents are making a big mistake when they allow their children unsupervised access to MTV. Many of the videos are riddled with satanic symbols if not outright portrayals of satanic obsession. Showing an interest in such evil allows Satan the opportunity to attach himself to your life, and once he establishes a beachhead, he is extremely difficult to remove.

Don't give him the opportunity in the first place!

11

........·.·.·...

VICTORY OVER WORRY

The world had never seen anything like the efficiency of the Roman legion. These men established a reputation as the consummate fighting machine largely because of their shoulder-to-shoulder fighting style. Prior to the triumph of Rome, men fought more as individuals than as a unit, but the Roman legionnaires attacked side-by-side in what were called phalanxes. Soon the phalanxes of the Roman legion became the terror of the ancient world as the soldiers marched shoulder-to-shoulder behind a solid wall of shields. As they marched, they struck their shields with their spears in unison and chanted their battle cries. Many an enemy fled in terror from the mere sound of their approach.

STATE-OF-THE-ART ARMOR

In addition to his tactical advantage, each legionnaire also enjoyed what was then considered state-of-the-art armor. Around his waist he wore a large, heavy belt which not only braced and supported him but also held his weapons. This freed both of his hands to wage combat.

To protect his vital organs, the legionnaire wore a metal breastplate. In those days prior to the discovery of gunpowder, the breastplate was capable of stopping any arrow or spear which the enemy could send his way.

The legionnaire's boots were heavy and had hobnails on the bottom to allow them to better grip the field or road during combat. Many an enemy was known to flee at the loud and frightening sound of thousands of hobnailed boots relentlessly marching toward them.

The fully armed legionnaire had a helmet to protect his head and a shield to shelter his body. The shield was large enough to

151

cover the soldier's entire body while he fearlessly brushed aside
the torrents of spears and arrows thrown his way.

Finally, each legionnaire carried the "Roman sword." It was
approximately two feet long, and unlike the Hun's sword, which
was sharpened only on the point, both sides of the Roman sword
were honed to razor sharpness. With this final weapon in his
arsenal, the legionnaire possessed an offensive weapon so deadly
that it overwhelmed the civilized world.

Rome remained the dominant world power longer than any
nation before or after largely because of the strength of its well-
armed warriors. When Rome finally lost its role as world leader,
it was more from internal decay than from a failure of its fighting
men.

GOD'S ELITE WARRIORS

But despite the formidable image cast by the Roman
legionnaire, he pales in comparison to the fully armed Christian
soldier. A brief study of the armor available to each and every
Christian reveals warriors capable of standing against Satan
himself. Hell itself shudders at the sight of God's elite warriors
marching shoulder-to-shoulder for the cause of Christ.

Ephesians 6:14–17 describes the Christian armor this way:
"Stand therefore, having girded your waist with truth, having
put on the breastplate of righteousness, and having shod your
feet with the preparation of the gospel of peace; above all, taking
the shield of faith, with which you will be able to quench all the
fiery darts of the wicked one. And take the helmet of salvation,
and the sword of the Spirit, which is the word of God."

When he is arrayed like this, there is no reason for the Christian
warrior to worry. Like the Roman soldier, the Christian can march
forward without worrying about his enemy, since he possesses
all the tools necessary for victory.

In this chapter we will learn how to outsmart the stresses that
can enter our lives when we allow worry to cloud our faith.
Ephesians 6:13 says that we are to stand against our enemy, not
to retreat. Worry is the cause of retreat: A soldier retreats when
his adversary has him worried. He doesn't believe he can
withstand the enemy's attack, and so he flees rather than stand
up to him. In the Christian life, worry occurs when a person
doesn't believe God's promises to care for him not only in battle,
but in every other aspect of daily life as well.

ARMED AND AWESOME

Although we face a dangerous foe, we are assured by God that we have all the armor necessary not only to withstand him but to gain a clear and decisive victory. Let's take a look at our arsenal.

1. *The belt of truth.* The first piece of armor mentioned in Ephesians 6:14 is the belt of truth. Like the Roman belt, it is foundational to hold the other weapons. The truth of God includes all of His promises to care for us. Armed with such knowledge, we are not vulnerable to the lies and deceit of our enemy, for we always know what the truth is.

   We are also assured that all of God's promises regarding His love for us are true, and that He wants only the best for those He loves. Armed with this fact, we should never worry about whether He has forsaken us. The fact that we can believe everything God has ever said is the foundation of true faith.

2. *The breastplate of righteousness.* We are told that Satan is the "accuser of the brethren," and yet God sees only our righteousness because of the work of His Son on the cross. Our souls are protected by the breastplate of righteousness.

3. *The boots of the gospel.* We are told in Ephesians 6:15 to protect our feet with the "preparation of the gospel of peace." The gospel is the good news that Jesus has established peace between God and man by paying for our sins on the cross. The good news is that we are no longer at war with God. We are now on the side of the omnipotent God of creation, and we need not fear the eventual outcome of the conflicts raging around us. Peace has been declared between Christians and their God.

4. *The shield of faith.* As the Roman soldier sought refuge under his mighty shield, the Christian soldier seeks protection from Satan's fiery darts under the shield of faith. Faith is the antithesis of worry.

   Some of Satan's most dangerous fiery darts are the darts of worry. Whereas faith is confidence in God's protection, love, and care, worry continually calls these into doubt. Not only is our salvation based on faith, but our successful daily walk must also be sheltered under the shield of faith in God's promises.

5. *The helmet of salvation.* Ephesians 6:17 warns us to cover our heads with the helmet of salvation. Even as our head is central to all we say, do, and think, likewise our salvation is the central feature of our Christian life. It is the unmistakable difference between God's children and all who stand against Him.

6. *The sword of the Spirit.* The elements of armor mentioned so far are basically defensive in nature and are used to ward off an attack by the enemy. The final tool in the Christian's arsenal is designed to be not only *defensive* but also *offensive.*

   The sword of the Spirit is defined in verse 17 as the Word of God. As a sword, it is used by the Christian both to ward off attacks by the enemy and to expand the kingdom of God. Used properly, it lodges in the mind of the hearer, and soon the Holy Spirit uses it to convict a person of his need for a Savior. More than just a book, the Bible is supernatural not only in its authorship, but also in the way in which it can break down the hardest of hearts through the work of the Holy Spirit.

THE CLOUD OF WORRY

But despite having access to such incredibly powerful weapons, many Christians live under what appears to be a cloud of worry. As stress builds in their lives, rather than attacking the source of their stress they retreat to a darkened corner to worry about the consequences. Not only does this fail to solve anything, but it is akin to throwing gasoline on the "stress fire." As Vance Havner observed, "Worry, like a rocking chair, will give you something to do, but it won't get you anywhere."

Many times we worry about things that are not worthy of our time, let alone our concern. They are like a cloud of fog which can appear to be incredibly thick but in fact contains hardly anything solid at all. Scientists tell us that a typical morning fog covering an area of seven square blocks to a depth of 100 feet may seem to contain lots of moisture, but in fact it is almost all air. It is composed of 60 trillion droplets of water so tiny that if all were brought together they would amount to less than one cup of water!

The cloud of worry at times appears totally impenetrable when in reality it is nothing more than air. Worry has been described as "the interest you pay on a debt you may never incur." People worry about things which might happen but in reality seldom do.

The University of Michigan did a study on the things people worry about and came to the conclusion that more than 97 percent of all worrying is a worthless waste of time. Their study found that:

60 percent of worries are totally unwarranted.

20 percent are past and unchangeable.

10 percent are too petty to waste your time on.

5 percent are unreal.

2 1/2 percent are real but you can't change them.

2 1/2 percent are real and worthy of worry.

In other words, 97 1/2 percent of the things people worry about aren't worth the time wasted on them! They may appear real, yet in most cases they are nothing but a dark cloud with very little substance.

But even though the *objects* of worry may not be real, the toll they extract from people is very real. Worry is the chief cause of the 10 million new cases of ulcers in America each year. Worry can lead to such agonies as migraine headaches, backaches, sexual impotence, high blood pressure, insomnia, poor grades, loss of friends, loss of jobs, and loss of Christian effectiveness. If it is not brought under control, worry will greatly increase the stress in your life. Let's take a look at how and why we can control worry.

STRANGLER ON THE LOOSE

While delivering the Sermon on the Mount, Jesus explicitly declared that we are not to worry. After His blanket prohibition of worry in Matthew 6:25, He supported His statement with several valid reasons. First His basic declaration: "Therefore I say to you do not worry about your life, what you will eat or what you will drink; nor about your body, what you will put on. Is not life more than food and the body more than clothing?"

Don't waste your time and energy worrying about the basics of life such as food, clothing, and shelter. God has promised to take care of these in the life of each believer, and He wants us focusing on loftier goals of service. A person obsessed with the fear of going hungry is of little use in spreading the good news of salvation. The German word for worry is *wurgen*, which means to strangle or choke. In a very real sense, worry serves to choke the flow of blessings in the life of a believer. One definition describes worry as "wasting today's time to clutter tomorrow's opportunities with yesterday's troubles." Worry has also been described as a stream of fear that runs through our mind. If we allow it to do so, it will cut a channel so wide that all our other thoughts will drown in it.

Worry is sin. Jesus clearly warned us not to worry, so to continue knowingly to worry is not only to disobey Him but also to call into doubt His promises to care for us. Recognizing the seriousness of worry, John Wesley used to say that he would just as soon swear as to worry. Worrying is evidence of a serious lack of trust in God and His unfailing promises. As E. E. Wordsworth elaborated, "Worry saddens, blights, destroys, kills. It depletes one's energies, devitalizes the physical man, and enervates the whole spiritual nature. It greatly reduces the spiritual stature and impoverishes the whole spirit."

WHY WE WORRY

Here are six major reasons why people waste their time and energies worrying. See if your favorite is on this list.

1. *Finances.* Few things get more "worry time" than personal finances. People worry about unpaid bills, the cost of putting kids through college, their inability to purchase a house, the lack of money to replace aging autos or appliances, and the possibility of being laid off or fired. Despite the fact that their income rises as people grow older, few ever reach a place where financial pressures no longer exist. It has never failed to amaze me how a family's expenses seem to increase at least as rapidly as their annual pay increases!

2. *Family.* The second major cause of worry centers around family relationships. Parents worry when their children become ill and when they struggle during their teen years. As their parents begin to experience the pain of aging, the children worry about their care. Wives worry whether their spouse is being unfaithful, and vice versa.

3. *Fatigue.* When people become fatigued, they are even more vulnerable to worry. Fatigue can either result from illness or lead to illness. In either case, worry can become a demoralizing affliction.

4. *Fear.* Different sciences have arisen dealing with specific fears experienced by various people. They range from a fear of spiders (arachnophobia) to a fear of tight spaces (claustrophobia). In addition to these widely recognized phobias are the basic human fears which we face daily, and which can cause painful worry. These include the fear of facing your angry boss, of meeting your girlfriend's parents, of having to speak in public, of not getting into a good college, of not having a date for the prom, or of becoming embarrassed in front of other people. Any of these fears can cause serious worry.

5. *Frustrations.* People worry about the things in life which cause them frustration, and the most frustrating problems are those which never seem to get resolved . . . they just linger on and on. When people find themselves in a difficult situation with no hope of relief in sight, their frustration is often accompanied by constant worry.

6. *Future.* Much worry centers around the uncertainty of the future. As they contemplate what the future will bring, some people see only the bad that could occur. In their minds they struggle over all the possible pain they may be forced to endure, when in fact things seldom turn out as bad as they worried about.

BIRDS WITHOUT WORRY

As Jesus stood on the lush and gentle slope of the hills ringing the north shore of the Sea of Galilee, He focused the attention of His listeners on the beauty of His Father's creation. For millennia this part of the Middle East has been a crossroads for birds migrating between the lands to the north and the winter feeding grounds in Africa. Jesus directed His hearers' attention to the wonder of the birds flying over them with His words in Matthew 6:26: "Look at the birds of the air, for they neither sow nor reap nor gather into barns; yet your heavenly Father feeds them. Are you not of more value than they?"

Jesus first reminded His listeners that birds don't waste their time worrying. And why should they? God has provided all they need. He not only created them but He sustains them. The fowl of the air can teach us much about living in the present without worrying about what the future may bring.

Martin Luther explained how a simple little bird taught him how to have victory over worry: "I have one preacher I love better than any other; it is my little tame robin, who preaches to me daily. I put his crumbs upon my windowsill, especially at night. He hops onto the sill when he wants his supply, and takes as much as he desires to satisfy his need. From there he always hops to a little tree close by, and lifts up his voice to God, and sings his carol of praise and gratitude, tucks his little head under his wings, and goes fast to sleep, to leave tomorrow to look after itself."

Of God's created beings, mankind stands alone in his propensity to worry about what he *doesn't* possess rather than to rejoice in what he *does* possess! No bird ever tried to build more nest than its neighbor. No fox ever fretted because he had only one hole in which to live and hide. No squirrel ever died of anxiety lest he fail to lay up enough nuts for two winters instead of one. No dog ever lost sleep over the fact that he did not have enough bones buried in the ground for his declining years. Animals are hard working members of God's creation, but so far as we know, they refuse to expend energy in the useless emotion of worry.

BETTER THAN BIRDS

In Matthew 6:26 Jesus asked His listeners, "Are you not of more value than they?" After all, if God cares so much for relatively unimportant creatures like the birds, consider how much He cares for *you*, His own child. The difference is extraordinary. In my house we had a bird named Pancho. We enjoyed him as a pet and made sure he was fed and protected from our cat and our six-year-old. But no matter how well I treated Pancho, he was never more than a pet. On an infinitely higher level are my five children. My love for them cannot be equated with my care of a bird. After all, they are my children.

If God takes care of something as relatively unimportant as a *bird*, imagine how He wants to take care of His *children*! Remember that God didn't send His only Son to die for the birds but rather for His children. Birds are not filled with the Holy Spirit, but His children are. Birds will not be adorned at the

Marriage Supper of the Lamb. Birds will not reign with Christ in eternity. If the birds have no need to worry, we as His *children* should not worry about whether He will provide for our daily needs. We are reminded of this point as Jesus continued in the Sermon on the Mount: "What man is there among you who, if his son asks for bread, will give him a stone? Or if he asks for a fish, will he give him a serpent? If you then, being evil, know how to give good gifts to your children, how much more will your Father who is in heaven give good things to those who ask Him!" (Matthew 7:9-11).

God has a reason for not wanting us to waste our time worrying about providing for life's basics: He knows there is something far more important for us to be seeking. This is stated in Matthew 6, when Jesus declared in verse 33, "But seek first the kingdom of God and His righteousness, and all these things shall be added to you." In this verse God promises that He will not fail to provide for our basic physical needs if we faithfully pursue a righteous life.

The result of such righteous living was observed nearly 3000 years ago by King David when he declared in Psalm 37:25, "I have been young, and now am old; yet I have not seen the righteous forsaken, nor his descendants begging bread." God didn't promise that He would make all of the righteous wealthy, but He did promise they would never be forsaken or have their offspring beg for food. I, like David 3000 years earlier, have never seen God forsake those who are truly righteous.

NO-GROWTH INVESTMENT

Matthew 6:27 reminds us that worrying is a most unproductive activity: "Which of you by worrying can add one cubit to his stature?" Most young boys experience anxious days as they begin to grow taller. They may be slow to hit their growth spurt, and so they suffer the agony of watching their friends grow a head taller than they are.

As their growth spurt strikes, their life may involve a daily ritual of measuring to see if they have caught up with their father or a close friend. Given an opportunity, most guys would choose to be a little taller than they are. But no matter how much a young man worries about being too short and no matter how often he worries about growing taller, it won't help him a bit, since worrying can't change a thing.

We learned that if God has taken such good care of the birds in the sky, He will certainly take better care of those of us who are His children. Now we are reminded that worry is a colossal waster of time. As we noted earlier, like rocking in a rocking chair, worry will give you something to do but certainly not get you anywhere. Time that could be invested in wholesome and productive thinking is used up by worrying about things beyond our control. As we noted earlier, God instructs us to pursue righteousness, and then He will take care of our basic needs.

Peter learned this lesson vividly in the classic story of his walking on the water. While the storm raged on the Sea of Galilee, Jesus told Peter to step out of the boat and walk across the water to Him. While the rest of the Twelve looked on in shock, Peter leaped out of the boat and with his eyes upon the Master walked toward Him on top of the water. As long as Peter obeyed Jesus in faith, God took care of his basic needs. It was only when Peter began to worry about those needs that he fell into trouble . . . and the water.

Worry is the flip side of faith. To worry about God's provision is to question His promises. As Jesus said with disappointment to Peter, "O you of little faith!"

LET TODAY BE TODAY

A third lesson about worry is found in Matthew 6:34: "Do not worry about tomorrow, for tomorrow will worry about its own things. Sufficient for the day is its own trouble." In other words, even though you may have to confront a difficult situation in the future, you do yourself no favor by ruining the present day worrying about it. You'll have plenty of time to deal with it when tomorrow comes.

I don't believe I've ever met a child (or adult, for that matter) who enjoys getting an inoculation shot. Recently my 11-year-old daughter learned that she would need to receive a shot later in the week. Despite our assurances, she spent the entire week in misery, dreading the coming pain. She actually suffered far more from worrying about the shot than from the actual pain of the shot! When the day finally arrived and she received her shot, she seemed surprised that it hurt as little as it did and was sorry she had ruined her week by worrying about it.

God gives a special type of sustaining grace to those who go through difficult crises. Many a Christian has marveled at how

God empowered him or her to endure what he previously would have considered unendurable. However, this special grace is given only when it is needed, and can seldom be drawn upon in advance to handle worry. Don't consume yourself worrying about what *might* happen in the future.

CROSSING THE FOX RIVER

Abraham Lincoln knew how to keep potential future disasters in the proper perspective. He learned early in his career not to worry about future problems. When Lincoln was on his way to Washington to be inaugurated as President, he spent some time in New York with Horace Greeley and told him an anecdote which was meant to be an answer to the question which everybody was asking him: Are we really ready for the Civil War? On one of his earlier circuit-riding days Lincoln and his companions, riding to the next session of court, had crossed several swollen rivers. But the Fox River was still ahead of them, and they said to one another, "If these streams give us so much trouble, how shall we get over the Fox River?"

Lincoln related, "When darkness fell, they stopped for the night at a log tavern, where they fell in with the Methodist presiding elder of the district, who rode through the country in all kinds of weather and knew all about the Fox River. They gathered around him and asked him about the present state of the river. 'I know all about the Fox River. I have crossed it often and understand it well. But I have one fixed rule with regard to the Fox River: I never cross it till I reach it.'"

The same advice applies to all of us and the uncertainties we face. To worry about them now is to waste God-given time and precious energy!

12

THE WINNING ATTITUDE

The story is told of how, through a long series of mistakes, the egg of a majestic eagle ended up in the nest of an American prairie chicken. Of course the eagle is known for its ability to soar through the sky as it searches out its prey, while the prairie chicken can neither fly nor hunt. Instead, it spends most of its time scratching in the dirt looking for insects to eat.

Before long the eggs all hatched and the young eaglet was taught to scratch in the dirt like any good prairie chicken. One afternoon he happened to glance up from his scratching and caught a glimpse of a powerful eagle soaring high on the thermals rising from the prairies. "Oh," he sighed to the other young prairie chickens, "I hope someday I'll be able to fly like that!"

With a tone of contempt in their voices they let him know he would never fly. "After all," they said, "you're just a prairie chicken." He knew they were right . . . he was just a prairie chicken, and everybody knew that prairie chickens can't fly. With a sense of resignation he lowered his head and went back to scratching for insects in the dirt.

What a sad and yet all-too-familiar story! Here was an eagle who had the power to fly with the mightiest of birds, yet he believed the others when they said he couldn't fly. He had an *attitude problem* which kept him scratching in the dirt.

THE JORDAN ATTITUDE

I am convinced of the power of *attitude* in changing a person's life. We will never accomplish any great feat in life until we convince ourselves that we can do it. Life is 10 percent what happens to us and 90 percent how we respond to what happens.

A skinny high school sophomore may take the news that he

has been cut from the high school basketball team as proof that he isn't quite good enough to play and should forget about the sport. It happens to young boys all the time. It also happened to Michael Jordan when he was a high school sophomore. The difference between him and the boys who gave up after hearing they had been cut was that Jordan knew he was good enough and set out to show his coach and the entire world what he knew about himself. Life is 10 percent getting cut from a sports team and 90 percent how you respond to it.

We see this clearly in events which can cause stress. The event itself is not nearly as important as *our attitude toward the event* when it comes to predicting how much stress will result. Let's look at how a positive and persistent attitude can be our greatest ally in outsmarting the inevitable stresses in our lives.

CONQUEST IN THE PEA PATCH

One of the major weaknesses that some people experience is the inability to remain focused on a goal. Success comes to those who clearly define their goals in life and funnel all their energies toward reaching those goals.

In 2 Samuel 23 we see some of King David's mighty men of valor. One of them, Shammah, is little-known and unmentioned elsewhere even though he stands as a monument to what can be achieved by a person who is totally focused on a single goal. The story is told briefly in 2 Samuel 23:11,12: "After him was Shammah the son of Agee the Hararite. The Philistines had gathered together into a troop where there was a piece of ground full of lentils. Then the people fled from the Philistines. But he stationed himself in the middle of the field, defended it, and killed the Philistines. And the Lord brought about a great victory."

There Shammah stood in the middle of what was really nothing more than a pea patch, alone against the enemies of God. He was willing to die defending what belonged to God's people. It didn't matter that the rest of the defenders fled; Shammah focused on his job and stood up to fight. By the time the dust had cleared, we read that "the Lord brought about a great victory" —all because one lone soldier focused all he had on his goal.

FIRE IN THE COLD

My first paid job in life involved delivering newspapers back home in Wyoming, Michigan. Some mornings I would be forced to make my rounds while the temperature had dropped to 15 degrees below zero. I clearly remember one such morning. As I was finishing my route, a friend met me as he was completing his. With the temperature still well below zero, we could not feel any heat from the sun, which had just risen above the horizon. From his pocket my friend produced a small magnifying glass and held it several inches above an extra newspaper he had. Within a matter of seconds, smoke and soon fire came from the spot on which he had focused the rays of the sun.

It didn't matter how cold it was; even though by themselves the rays of the sun seemed to generate little energy, when properly focused toward the goal the energy was sufficient to create light, heat, and fire.

We need to think about the power of a focused life and what can result from it. Often a leader is needed to focus the energies of many different people toward the accomplishment of a single goal. By themselves the people would have little impact, but when directed toward the same precise target, they ignite a fire. This can occur in a church when a body of believers combine their spiritual gifts and energies to light a great fire for Christ.

On some occasions one person (such as Shammah) is asked to stand alone in a great undertaking. The key to victory is not in the number of people focused but in the *persistence of the personal focus*. Shammah refused to quit until the victory had been won.

PERSIST AND WIN

Few things are more stressful than failure. I hate to fail at anything, and I know I am not alone in this feeling. I am convinced that one of the most common causes of failure is that people give up just before the victory is achieved. They lack the all-important attitude of *persistence* and are subsequently stressed out by their lack of success in life.

The book of Ephesians closes with a call to persistence. It reminds us that the battles in life are seldom won by the "morning glories," but by those with the attitude of persistence in the face of resistance.

After commanding the Christian warrior to stand up to Satan and not to flee, God instructs us to don the entire armor He has made available for our defense. Despite cautioning us about the ruthless power of the adversary, God encourages us with the good news that victory can be ours if we put on the whole armor and resolutely stand against the devil.

Unfortunately, many Christians make it this far, only to fail because they neglect to heed the verses which follow. Ephesians 6:18-20 warns, "praying always with all prayer and supplication in the Spirit, being watchful to this end with all perseverance and supplication for all the saints—and for me, that utterance may be given to me, that I may open my mouth boldly to make known the mystery of the gospel, for which I am an ambassador in chains; that in it I may speak boldly, as I ought to speak."

THE UNSHEATHED SWORD

The key to victory is found in verse 18. It is not enough merely to put on all the armor; we must keep it on! Far too many Christians quit the battles of life before they are over, and end up frustrated. Verse 18 talks about persistent prayer. Most Christians are quick to heed the call to present their needs to the Lord in prayer but tend to tire if the desired response does not come quickly. Throughout Scripture we are told that it is the "effective fervent prayer" which avails much. A fervent intercessor will continue to bring his petitions to the Lord and not tire easily.

In verse 18 the Christian soldier is told to be constantly watchful, to keep his armor on and his sword unsheathed until his days on earth are done. We are told to do it "with all perseverance," for it is *persistence* which wins battles. To quit a battle while still in the presence of the enemy is a sure way to bring additional stress into your life. No soldier should enter a battle unless he is prepared to see it through to the end. His preparation must begin by developing an attitude of persistence, to settle in his mind that nothing short of finishing the battle is acceptable.

NOT BRAINS BUT GUTS

Although himself a brilliant man, when Theodore Roosevelt was asked about the key to success in life, he proclaimed that it is not the I.Q. but rather the "I WILL" that most determines a person's relative success in life. He was a firm believer in the value of learning from failures as well as successes in molding character. Others have pointed out that genius has very little to do with success. This helps to explain why all of us remember kids with whom we attended school who were considered the "class brains," and yet years later we discover that they failed to cash in on their intellectual advantage.

Many times when things come easily to a person, he or she never learns the importance of the struggle. He doesn't know how to overcome a failure because he has never before faced one.

Some young boys are taller than their friends and have little trouble making the high school basketball team, yet they never learn to work hard and master the fundamentals of the game. They do all right in high school because they are taller than most of the other players, but they receive a rude awakening if they try to play college basketball. At this point they discover that the league is filled with young men who are equally tall but who have also been working for years on the fundamentals of the game.

A LIFE OF FAILURE?

Sometimes an apparent advantage can turn into a potential liability. This may be what prompted Immanuel Kant to remark, "I have never seen a precocious child amount to much as an adult." Such children all too often miss the lessons to be learned in the "School of Hard Knocks."

Remember, it isn't the failure that matters nearly so much as how you respond to it. Consider the case of the young businessman who, after watching his new business fail, decided to run for the state legislature but was defeated in his bid for office. With no way to support himself, he went back into business, but to his disappointment he saw this endeavor fail as well.

Shortly after this disappointment he was crushed by the death of his sweetheart. These events combined to cause him a nervous breakdown the following year. Two years later he again sought public office as state speaker, but as before, he suffered defeat. In addition, he was defeated in his bids for both the state house and the U.S. Congress during the five years which followed.

After all these defeats and failures, he was finally elected to the U.S. Congress. It may have appeared as if his career was at last on track, but this dream was crushed when two years later he was rejected in his bid for reelection. The failures seemed to multiply as he was defeated in his bid for the U.S. Senate seven years later, the vice-presidency a year after that, and finally the U.S. Senate one last time two years later.

What a life of failure! After suffering eight defeats in bids for public office, who would have thought that two years later Abraham Lincoln would be elected President of the United States of America! Probably no one alive at that time would have thought so except Abraham Lincoln . . . and he never had any doubts. The apparent failures were nothing more than part of his learning process. They were what prepared him to lead this nation through its darkest hour, for he was now a uniquely qualified leader.

THE TEN-MILLION-DOLLAR EDUCATION

Thomas Watson, the president of IBM, used to say, "If you want to double your success rate, double your failure rate." This philosophy is shown in the true story about a project manager at IBM who had just lost the company 10 million dollars. He had his resignation in hand as he walked into the president's office and said, "I'm sorry. I'm sure you'll want my resignation. I'll be gone by the end of the day."

The president's response showed his understanding of the value of failure when he replied, "Are you kidding? We've just invested 10 million dollars in your education. We're not about to let you go. Now get back to work."

Most people are not aware that Thomas Edison failed almost 8000 times before he got it right in inventing the light bulb. That's how many different filaments he burned up in his quest to find the proper material. When asked how he felt about all the failures, the great genius replied simply, "They weren't failures, they were education."

Unfortunately, the fear of failing can keep many people from even attempting to reach their goal. They literally give up before they ever start. It takes courage to start a challenge, but once started it seldom seems as frightening anymore. It's the getting started that can be so difficult. Woody Allen remarked that 80 percent of success is just showing up.

Starting a difficult task is a bit like pushing a locomotive. When it is at rest, several small blocks of wood strategically placed underneath its wheels will keep it from moving even though its engines are revved up. Even with the blocks removed, it takes tremendous energy and time for the heavy locomotive to gain speed. However, once it gains speed and momentum, it will take tons of reinforced concrete just to slow it down.

The key is not only getting started, but getting started now. Don't put it off or there is an excellent chance the challenge will never see the light of day. As someone has said, "If you don't get started in the next 72 hours, you ain't gonna get started at all."

THE IMPOSSIBLE CHAMPION

Many people stop pursuing their goal because of the apparent obstacles that lie before them. In any worthy quest, formidable obstacles will arise to discourage all but the most persistent people from achieving success. Those who press on usually benefit greatly from the process as well as the results.

In 1962, Victor and Mildred Goertzel published *Cradles of Eminence*, which is a revealing analysis of 413 famous and exceptionally gifted people. Their goal was to identify common elements in the lives of these exceptional people which might have produced their greatness. To their surprise, the most outstanding fact was that 392 of the 413 people had to overcome very difficult obstacles in order to achieve their greatness. Rather than preventing their greatness, the obstacles forced these people to develop persistence and thereby to achieve their greatness.

In the early days of this century, a pair of ten-year-old boys accidentally poured gasoline instead of kerosene on a stove fire in their little country schoolhouse. The resulting explosion killed one of the boys instantly and injured the legs of his friend so badly that his doctors recommended amputation.

Because of the pleading of the boy's parents, the doctors kept delaying the amputation until, after several months, they decided that the boy's legs might be saved after all. When the bandages were removed, they discovered legs that could never again be used for walking. The right leg was 2 1/2 inches shorter than the left leg, and the right foot was missing most of its toes.

With burning determination, the boy learned how to walk again, first with crutches, and then painfully without crutches. One day he actually broke into a wobbly jog, but he was determined to do better . . . much better. And better he did. Within a handful of years this boy, Glenn Cunningham, had become one of the greatest runners in Olympic history. In fact, he was once called "the world's fastest human being."

In the case of Glenn Cunningham, rather than preventing him

from achieving greatness, the obstacles he faced actually helped him to become great, because he found the secret of *persisting despite obstacles.*

In this adaptation from Paul Speiker consider some of the obstacles which have forged greatness:

> Cripple him, and you have a Sir Walter Scott.
>
> Lock him in a prison cell, and you have a John Bunyan.
>
> Bury him in the snows of Valley Forge, and you have a George Washington.
>
> Subject him to bitter religious prejudice, and you have a Disraeli.
>
> Afflict him with asthma as a child, and you have a Theodore Roosevelt.
>
> Stab him with rheumatic pains until he can't sleep without an opiate, and you have a Steinmetz.
>
> Put him in a grease pit of a locomotive roundhouse, and you have a Walter P. Chrysler.
>
> Make him second fiddle in an obscure South American orchestra, and you have a Toscanini.
>
> At birth, deny a child the ability to see, hear, and speak, and you have a Helen Keller.

CLOSING THE PATENT OFFICE

Many people shy away from situations that contain high levels of risk, while others seem to enjoy the adrenaline rush that comes from having their well-being in jeopardy. Risk can involve more than placing your life in danger; it can just as easily include trying to achieve something never before tried, or taking on a job with no reward unless you achieve success.

A basic rule is *the higher the risk, the greater the possible reward.* This was shown dramatically in a survey of the 1985 earnings of professional salesmen from 750 U.S. sales organizations. The researchers discovered that salesmen working with some form of guaranteed salary earned a respectable average of $47,700 in 1985. They then calculated the average earnings of the 6.4 percent of the salesmen from these 750 companies who were willing to work without a safety net. Working on a commission-only basis, they didn't earn anything if they didn't sell anything. The results were startling: The average salesman in *this* group of risk-takers earned $185,600 during the same year of 1985!

Risk-taking involves believing that not all the good ideas have yet been thought up, and that your ideas have merit. Much of the world is suspicious of anything new or innovative and will refuse to try something unless it has already been proven to work.

In 1899 a letter was sent to the President of the United States by the director of the U.S. Office of Patents. After watching all the great innovations of the industrial revolution, he was convinced that everything worth inventing had already been invented, so he recommended permanently shutting down the U.S. Office of Patents!

With technology virtually exploding before our very eyes, I'm convinced that some of man's most creative moments lie just ahead of us. Don't fear to risk an attempt merely because something like this has never before been done. Don't be a slave to the experts who are quick to discourage flights into the unknown.

FASTER THAN FOUR?

In 1945, Gunder Haegg ran the mile faster than any human being had ever run it, with a time of 4:01.4. As the sports experts considered this feat, they repeated what the experts had said for years: It was physically impossible for a human being to run the mile in less than four minutes.

And it appeared they were right, at least in 1946, 1947, 1948, 1949, etc. Gunder Haegg's time of 4:01.4 seemed to be the fastest the human body could endure.

However, a young British runner by the name of Roger Bannister failed to heed the advice of the experts. In 1954 Roger Bannister broke the tape at the end of a mile at 3:59.4!

The sports world was shocked, not only by Bannister's effort, but by the assault that followed. Now convinced that the "impossible barrier" had been shattered, in almost no time the four-minute achievement was bettered 66 times by 26 different men! They were just waiting for someone to prove that the goal was possible.

Learn the thrill of attempting what has not yet been proven. Learn of the rewards which come to those who refuse to be discouraged by so-called experts, and are willing to take risks . . . to work without a safety net.

DISCOURAGED BY BULLFROGS?

Whenever a person steps out of the line of mediocrity in which the rest of the world marches, the first sound to reach their hearing will be that of criticism. This is especially true if he or she assumes a position of leadership. No matter how well-liked or competent a leader may be, he will still suffer the fiery darts of criticism. I'm sure that's what prompted President Harry S. Truman to warn, "If you can't stand the heat, stay out of the kitchen."

The fear of criticism has caused many potential leaders to fall short of their potential. According to James Schorr of Holiday Inns, "Some of the most talented people are terrible leaders because they have a crippling need to be loved by everyone." They refuse to make decisions which might cause them to be criticized.

Criticism usually emanates from a small but vocal group of individuals. After I had spent several years at my church, I learned that if there was criticism of something we had initiated, it almost always came from the same three people. They were the kind of people who would criticize penicillin! More than once when a concerned staff member shared that "a number of people are unhappy with . . . " I startled him by naming the individuals. I soon learned that criticism from these people should never influence my course of action. They were a lot like the story of the bullfrog.

For years a farmer had each evening endured the noise from his "bullfrog pond." Finally deciding he could tolerate the racket and croaking no longer, he determined to drain the bullfrog pond and feast on an ample supply of fresh frog legs. As the level of the water dropped, the farmer made a fascinating discovery: Sitting and croaking on the muddy bottom of the pond was one solitary and indignant bullfrog!

Many times one old bullfrog is responsible for most of the criticism you hear. Don't be quick to alter your mission simply because you hear a lot of croaking. It may all be coming from one very active bullfrog.

Experience has taught me that time invested in answering your critics is usually time wasted. Be quick to heed valid and constructive criticism, but don't become obsessed in answering the bullfrogs and the naysayers. It is far better to invest that time in successfully completing your goal.

BUILD YOUR CANAL

Colonel George Washington Goethals felt the sting of criticism when he agreed to lead the latest U.S. effort to build what we now know as the Panama Canal. In light of the earlier disastrous attempts by both the French and the Americans, many were the pessimists who criticized Goethal's unusual scheme to carve a canal across the malaria-infested swamps of the Isthmus of Panama. Goethals had to endure the carping criticism of countless busybodies back home who freely predicted that he would never complete his project. But he pressed forward steadily in his work and said nothing.

"Aren't you going to answer your critics?" a friend once asked.

"In time," Goethals replied.

"How?" asked his friend.

"With the canal," Goethals replied.

When people criticize you, the best way to defend yourself is to prove them wrong "with the canal." The successfully completed project will stand as irrefutable evidence that your critics were wrong. If, on the other hand, you fail to "build the canal," your critics will be proven right and your personal defense will appear foolish. Just build your canal. It's the best way to silence your critics.

NEVER GIVE UP!

Winston Churchill probably understood the value of persistence better than most men who have ever lived. A study of his life reveals a man who was forever failing on a scale that brought upon him the scorn of his critics, and yet as the twentieth century draws to a close, many people would consider him the most important and influential man of our century. Churchill had a rare talent for turning failure into success through perseverance.

After his heroic leadership in World War Two, Churchill was invited to speak at a prep school where he had been considered quite a failure while a student there. As the headmaster introduced this man who was now recognized as one of the greatest orators of all time, he instructed the room full of schoolboys to "be sure you take copious notes, because this will probably be one of the greatest speeches you'll ever hear."

As Churchill made his way to the podium and fixed his gaze on the eager faces in the crowded auditorium, he declared, "Never give up!" After a brief pause he caught his breath and continued even more boldly: "NEVER give up!" Another pause followed, and then, pounding his fist on the lectern, he shouted at the top of his lungs: "Never, never, NEVER GIVE UP!"

With those three words Winston Churchill captured the secret to succeeding in life: Never give up despite failures, obstacles, risks, or criticism. Use the winds of stress to propel you to greater achievement in all you do. View life's challenges as opportunities rather than obstacles, and you will truly conquer the stresses of life!

BIBLIOGRAPHY

_____. *An Introduction to Stress.* Life Skills Education, Inc., March, 1986.

"City Stress Index." *Psychology Today,* November, 1988.

Coping with Stress. Hartford, Connecticut: Keywood Publications, Inc., July, 1983.

"Coping with Stress." *Parents.* February, 1989.

Criswell, W. A. *Ephesians.* Grand Rapids, Michigan: Zondervan Publishing House, 1974.

"Dealing with Job Change." *Changing Times,* April, 1988.

Dickason, C. Fred. *Angels, Elect and Evil.* Chicago: Moody Press, 1975.

Dobson, James C. *Parenting Isn't for Cowards.* Word Books Publishers: Waco, Texas, 1987.

"Exercise Is the Key to Keeping Pounds Off." *USA Today,* January 2, 1991.

_____. *Family Finances,* Newhall, California: Stewardship Services Foundation, 1992.

"Five Ways to Fight Family Stress." *Reader's Digest,* February, 1987.

Gossett, Don. *How to Cope When You Can't.* Lafayette, Louisiana: Huntington House, Inc., 1986.

Hodge, Charles. *Commentary on the Epistle to the Ephesians.* Old Tappan, New Jersey: Fleming H. Revell Company.

Iaccoca, Lee. *Iaccoca*. New York: Bantam Books, 1984.

Jeremiah, David. *Before It's Too Late*. Nashville: Thomas Nelson Publishers, 1983.

LaHaye, Tim. *How to Be Happy Though Married*. Wheaton, Illinois: Tyndale House Publishers, Inc., 1983.

_____. *How to Manage Pressure Before Pressure Manages You*. Grand Rapids, Michigan: Zondervan Publishing House, 1983.

_____. *The Battle for the Family*. Old Tappan, New Jersey: Fleming H. Revell Company, 1982.

MacArthur, John Jr. *The MacArthur New Testament Commentary . . . Ephesians*. Chicago: Moody Press, 1986.

_____. *Your Family*. Chicago: Moody Press, 1982.

MacDonald, Gordon. *Magnificent Marriage*. Wheaton, Illinois: Tyndale House Publishers, Inc., 1983.

_____. *The Effective Father*. Wheaton, Illinois: Tyndale House Publishers, Inc., 1983.

"Managing Stress and Living Longer." *USA Today Periodical*, May, 1990.

Mead, Frank S., ed., *The Encyclopedia of Religious Quotations*. Old Tappan, New Jersey: Fleming H. Revell Company, 1965.

Montgomery, John Warwick. *Principalities and Powers*. Minneapolis, Minnesota: Bethany Fellowship, 1981.

Ogilvie, Lloyd J. *Making Stress Work for You*. Waco, Texas: Word Books Publishers, 1985.

Peretti, Frank E. *This Present Darkness*. Westchester, Illinois: Good News Publishers, 1986.

Peters, Thomas J., and Waterman, Robert H. Jr. *In Search of Excellence*. New York: Warner Books, Inc., 1984.

"Points to Ponder." *Reader's Digest*, January, 1991.

"School Stress Signals." *Parents*, October, 1988.

Schuller, Robert H. *Tough Times Never Last, But Tough People Do!* Nashville: Thomas Nelson Publishers, 1983.

_____. *Turning Your Stress into Strength*. Eugene, Oregon: Harvest House Publishers, 1978.

Sehnert, Keith W. *Stress/Unstress*. Minneapolis, Minnesota: Augsburg Publishing House, 1981.

Selye, Hans. *The Stress of Life*. New York: McGraw-Hill Book Company, 1978.

_____. *Stress and Your Child*. South Deerfield, Massachusetts: Channing L. Bete Company, Inc., 1987.

"Stress on the Job." *Newsweek*, April 25, 1988.

Swindoll, Charles R. *Stress Fractures*. Portland, Oregon: Multnomah Press, 1990.

Tan, Paul Lee. *Encyclopedia of 7700 Illustrations*. Rockville, Maryland: Assurance Publishers, 1980.

"Ten Ways to Master Stress Before It Masters You." *Virtue*, September/October, 1989.

"Thirty-nine Ways to Destress Your Home Life." *Prevention*, September, 1987.

"To Beat Stress, Don't Relax: Get Tough." *Psychology Today*, December, 1989.

Tozer, A. W. *Root of the Righteous*. Harrisburg: Christian Publications, Inc., 1955.

"Turning Stress Into Profit." *Macleans*, June 1, 1987.

"What Makes Kids Feel Bad?" *Ladies' Home Journal*, August, 1988.

Whitehead, John W. *The Stealing of America*. Westchester, Illinois: Crossway Books, 1983.

_____. *Who's Who in U.S. High Schools*. Poll of Students, 1980.

SCRIPTURE INDEX